KETO MADE EASY
THE 7 DAY AIR FRYER Challenge

Automate Your Keto Diet, Lose Stubborn Belly Fat, and Feel Great at Any Age!

Evan Harmelink

www.EvanHabits.com

CONTENTS

Introduction: Food for thought 9

1. Keto Diet Confusion 15
2. Too Many Daily Decisions with Our Food and Drink 33
3. Our Fuel Source is Wrong 39
4. Setting Goals but with No Vehicle for Action 65
5. Weekly Meal Prep is too Complex 81
6. Your Simple 7 Day Recipes 93
7. Challenge Checklist for Success 115

References 139

"This book is dedicated to you, the unsung heroes in real life. The struggle is real. Change is hard. You choose resilience in the face of adversity and then take action to improve."

YOUR FREE GIFT

To express my gratitude for purchasing my book and taking action on looking and feeling better with this Keto Challenge, here is a tasty reward! **My "Top 5 Keto Comfort Food Swap Recipes."** The Challenge Community upvoted these recipes, which can be accessed by clicking the link below. You don't need to sacrifice your favorite foods to improve your health when following the Keto Lifestyle. I think you will love these recipes as much as we have over the years. *My favorite is the pizza... or is it the chili?!*

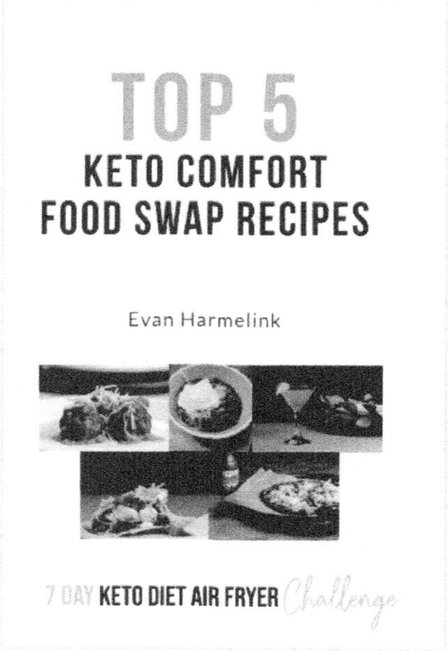

Grab your free recipes here:**_https://evanhabits.com/free-recipes/**

You can use your camera's phone to scan the Q.R. code below to go right to it as well.

INTRODUCTION: FOOD FOR THOUGHT

Keto may not be for everyone, but cutting down on processed, sugary foods absolutely is.

I wrote this book for you because I firmly believe that Keto is worth trying, or trying again, for almost everyone for a period of time. Many can even make it a *lifestyle*. This Challenge is your opportunity to test drive Keto the easy way, with a dietary G.P.S., removing all food-based decisions and automating that you arrive at your desired destination—*eating Keto. This book automates cutting out the high levels of sugar—another word for simple carbohydrate—and as a result, you will be successfully eating Keto in just seven days.*

If you live in the U.S.A., by default, chances are excellent that you are eating what is known as the Standard American Diet, *or S.A.D.* There are many variations, but to boil it down in the simplest of terms, the S.A.D. is this: Eating lots of carbohydrates, an average of 200 to 300 grams per day, with many of those foods highly processed. This is exactly what keeps 73.1 percent of the American adult population overweight, obese, or even, **gasp** extremely obese. *This is very S.A.D. indeed (pun intended).*

The majority of adults twenty years old and older in the U.S. are fat and sick. The diet the majority of us are eating is not working. It's time to do something radically different if we expect different results! Keto is that *something*!

Does Keto work? Don't just take my word for it (a marketer selling a book on the internet) ... Over many years, there have been published studies that confirm very positive outcomes for people that eat the Keto Diet, for weight loss, and much more.

Here are the combined results of 66 published studies on Keto and weight loss alone:

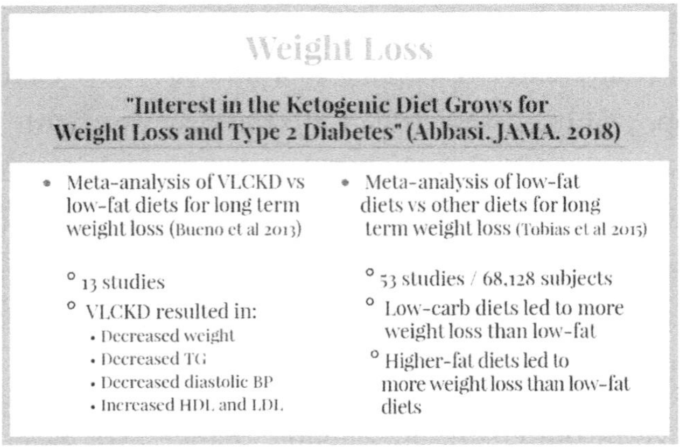

Weight Loss
"Interest in the Ketogenic Diet Grows for Weight Loss and Type 2 Diabetes" (Abbasi. JAMA. 2018)
Meta-analysis of VLCKD vs low-fat diets for long term weight loss (Bueno et al 2013)
13 studies
VLCKD resulted in:
Decreased weight
Decreased TG
Decreased diastolic BP
Increased HDL and LDL
Meta-analysis of low-fat diets vs other diets for long term weight loss (Tobias et al 2015)
53 studies / 68,128 subjects
Low-carb diets led to more weight loss than low-fat
Higher-fat diets led to more weight loss than low-fat diets

Yes, Keto has been proven to help many of us lose fat effectively, but it has not always been easy to execute. *It can be too hard.* In fact, many versions you may have seen or tried are ridiculously hard to sustain for any length of time. It's a huge issue. My Challenge when creating this course for you was: *How could I get you, my friend, to try Keto—or maybe try it again—and make it so simple that your results were guaranteed?* It had to be a no-brainer. I felt I needed to come up with the *Minimum Effective Keto Diet.* It had to be the easiest version of the Keto Diet that has ever been put in a book or an online course. Mission accomplished! This easy-to-follow 7 Day Air Fryer Challenge will remove all food-based decisions and will not require any discipline at all.

In the pages ahead, I've distilled down what I believe to be the five main reasons all diets fail, including the Keto Diet. I will expose and then remove these pitfalls for you with my simple habit system that will automate eating Keto for you.

Top Five Reasons Diets Fail (including Keto)

- **Reason #1:** Keto diet confusion... too much information creating "*paralysis by analysis*"
- **Reason #2:** Too many daily decisions with our food and drinks... our willpower runs out
- **Reason #3:** Our fuel source is wrong... sugar is a drug keeping us fat and sick
- **Reason #4:** Setting goals... but with no vehicle for action
- **Reason #5:** Weekly meal prep is too complex... too expensive... too time consuming

These five reasons diets fail have a HUGE impact on keeping us fat and sick as a nation. I will include information in a chapter devoted to each of these five reasons, as awareness is power. This 7 Day Keto Diet Air Fryer Challenge will allow you to sidestep all these reasons, so you can finally get the results you are looking for! The key to achieving results is the one-two punch of *awareness and action.* I'm serving you up the awareness and the plan for consistent action right here!

If you don't have a set of habits to guarantee eating a specific way, you won't.

Just like our goals, all the information in the world is useless if you don't take systematic actions to guarantee your results. You need to *do* the thing, not just think about it. This 7 Day Challenge will automate for you to reach your Keto eating goals.

Why the air fryer?

The air fryer checks all the boxes for the Minimum Effective Keto Diet:

- ☑ **No cooking skills needed**
- ☑ **Affordable**
- ☑ **Less time needed**
- ☑ **Healthy cooking technique**
- ☑ **Delicious food**
- ☑ **Effortless cleanup**

It's true with the air fryer!! The air fryer is a compact size convection heat oven that anyone can use anywhere you have an electric outlet and two square feet of counter space. Less really can be more.

How to eat Keto does not have to be confusing. The recipes don't have to be complex. It does not have to be expensive or hard at all.

It won't be any of these things here.

The habit of how we fuel our bodies is a game changer and impacts every area of our lives, for better or for worse. In this 7 Day Challenge, you will have a personal Keto eating system that will reduce your daily decision fatigue and make your willpower *automatic*. Just seven days following this outline will give you *Keto momentum* and is the beginning of a powerful, sustainable, life-changing habit for you and your loved ones. You will always have the answer to this daily question:

"What am I going to eat today?"

I hear way too many people give up and just accept feeling like garbage based on their biological age. It doesn't have to be that way for us! Age really is just a number, and it alone should not dictate how we feel. I'm fifty-three, and I can tell you after upgrading my fuel source from sugar to fat, I look and feel better now than when I was in my early twenties. It's never too late to improve how you look and feel. The "how to" is all done for you in the simple challenge outline ahead.

You can start this week! Congratulations on investing in YOU!

1

KETO DIET CONFUSION

Keto Confused?! Trust me, you are not alone. Maybe you have been at least "Keto curious" in the past? Maybe you jumped on Amazon and bought the books or scoured multitudes of keto YouTube videos to gather all the information? Maybe you jumped on social media and searched hundreds of Keto recipes to help you do Keto, then ... no action. Or some action *but no traction.* Paralysis by analysis set in yet again. Changing your eating habits just became too hard again. Change is not easy, but it's necessary to get the results you are looking for. *Change is not always easy, but it can be simple.*

The Keto Diet, or any diet, can be too hard to actually stick to in real life. The complex Keto definitions everywhere and the many opinions from so-called "trusted sources" do not help. When you add the complex, sixteen-plus ingredient recipes to the mix that take hours to prepare, you are ready to quit before you even start. We can't forget to mention here the many complicated counting and tracking apps designed to *help* us organize all the confusing data. It's all a bit much, right? It's understandable why most people may believe that dieting, especially Keto, is way too hard and that they give up before getting any lasting results!

If you do a quick "Keto Diet" Google search, here are a few of the variations of Keto you will find (and there are many more).

Standard Ketogenic Diet (S.K.D.), Modified Ketogenic Diet (M.K.D.), Cyclical Ketogenic Diet (CKD), Targeted Ketogenic Diet (T.K.D.), Restricted Ketogenic Diet (R.K.D.), High Protein Ketogenic Diet (H.P.K.D.), Vegan/Vegetarian Ketogenic Diet, Dirty/Clean Keto Diet, Keto 2.0, 3.0, etc., Lazy Keto Diet, Mediterranean Keto Diet, Atkins Diet, South Beach Diet, Low Carb High Fat Diet (L.C.H.F.), Paleo Diet, Low Glycemic Index Diet.

These many different—and often confusing—versions of Keto can all get out of hand and are not necessary to execute a healthy Keto lifestyle and to see and feel significant results. In the simplest terms, a Keto Diet comes down to JUST ONE THING:

A daily carb limit for your food intake

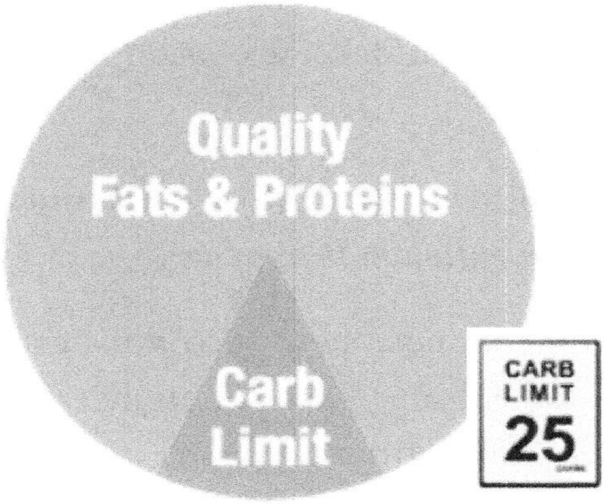

Limiting your daily carb intake directs your body to change its main fuel source from sugar to fat. *That's it.* Nothing more complex than that... *call it whatever you want.*

Isn't Keto just another fad diet?

In a word, no. The Keto Diet has been around for a very long time. This way of eating has been around for over 100 years and counting. It's not going away. It's been used as a successful medical intervention for conditions like childhood epilepsy. Again, there are decades of data at this point showing that eating Keto can successfully reduce our body fat. The Keto Diet, or some version of it, has gone up and down and up again in popularity over many decades. It keeps coming back because it works for many. Many best-selling books about eating low-carb have been written over the years. *The Atkins Diet* and *The*

South Beach Diet are just two that I purchased and read years ago. My dad got the first Atkins diet book published and had great success losing weight following the guidelines in the book. Yep, eating lots of delicious bacon helped my dad drop the pounds!

Let's get one thing straight right now: *Obesity is a disease that needs dietary intervention in this country.*

It truly makes me wonder how such a historically successful diet continues to be dismissed, or not fully embraced, by many more of our so-called trusted sources. The data has been published, and the time has passed. The real-life success stories are all there. Check, check, check. It's a real head-scratcher, for sure. I'm completely baffled at this point.

Many health and wellness professionals still refuse to recommend it to their clients or patients to this day, in 2023, even as a short-term weight loss intervention tool. I agree, it can be too hard to execute if it's made too confusing or complex. *But* it works for many if and when it is followed, so how about we ask a better question? How about instead, we ask how we can make it so easy that anyone can do it? As you will see in this course, I've done that for you! Keep it simple, stupid.

I have seen plenty of other reasons for its dismissal, like, "We still have not seen long-term evidence of it being effective..." Yet, plenty of published studies exist, and plenty of time has passed, with millions of people experiencing great results. I'd say 100-plus years and multitudes of studies with successful weight loss outcomes for humans really *should* be enough to consider trying Keto. Yes, it's time for you to try it and see if this can be effective for you, right?

The Standard American Fad (read Fat) Diet

In fact, the Standard American Diet of today is more of a *fad diet* than the Keto Diet is. This insidious S.A.D. fad crept into our culture over seventy years ago. The S.A.D. has been entrenched ever since and has been directly contributing to our obesity epidemic in this country. Old teachings, outdated beliefs, and bad eating habits have proven to die hard. Change is not easy. It's human nature to have a hard time admitting that we were wrong about anything and an even harder time apologizing for it and course-correcting. Most people, including health professionals, used to believe that cigarette smoking was not a serious health hazard, either. As you will see in the pages ahead, plenty of manipulation strategies are at play, driven by profits, that are keeping us fat and sick.

Too much information can make us stupid

> Angelika Dimoka, Director of The Center for Neural Decision Making at Temple University, conducted studies to see what happens when people's decision-making abilities are overtaxed. She found rational and logical prefrontal cortex functioning declined when it became overloaded with information, and as a result, subjects in her experiments began to make stupid mistakes and bad

choices. ***"With too much information," says Dimoka, "people's decisions make less and less sense."***

Confusing Keto Diet macros, blah, blah, blah...

Some Keto books and apps will advise you to consume each of these macronutrients as a percentage of the total calories consumed. For me, "percentages of other things" explanations become complex and way too confusing. An example would be the goal of eating 20 percent of my daily intake of protein, 70 percent of fat, and 10 percent of carbs. *Do I need a digital food scale in my home and car when I travel to figure this out? How about an Excel spreadsheet to track these macro percentages per meal? What does this actually look like on my plate, and how do I make all this?* Let's take a hard pass on all that complex tracking stuff; it's one of the huge reasons the Keto Diet is too hard and, therefore, not sustainable.

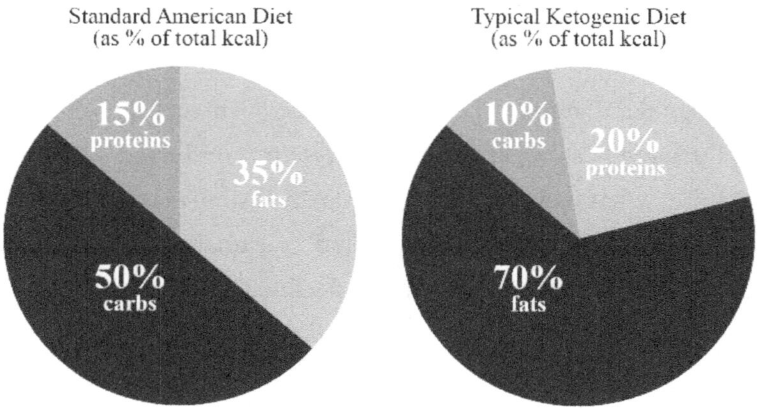

The simple version of Keto you will see HERE: *A set daily carb limit for your food intake.*

That's it, *very simple.* To make the shift to burning fat for your fuel source instead of sugar, we need to limit the carbs that we consume per day. That's all done for you with the daily recipes for your Challenge. You don't need to count or track anything on your 7 Day Challenge. You can't eat too much or too little protein or fat... just eat till you are full according to the menu for the week ahead.

***What are we NOT going to eat on Keto?* A high amount of refined, processed carbohydrates.**

The average adult American consumes 200 to 300 Grams of carbohydrates per day and many of them are highly processed. This recommendation comes directly from our government and many other "trusted sources.". This eating pattern is code for the Standard American Diet. It's code for diseases, too. Sugar is interchangeable with carbohydrates. When consumed, the body converts it into glucose. Insulin does not care what form of sugar enters the body (cane sugar or an apple). Its job is to remove the excess sugar (converted to glucose) from the bloodstream. Some sugar in the form of glucose is used for energy, and the unused portions go into fat cells and usually stay there for a long time. *In short, the S.A.D. is a recipe for obesity.*

Now, all foods containing carbs are not created equally dreadful. There are levels of dreadful... real, whole foods—like an apple, for example—contain some healthy micronutrients and fiber that are indeed good for us. But when all forms of carbohydrates are digested, they do turn into lower-grade fuel for the body and brain. I will refer to this lower-grade fuel source as burning sugar for fuel. This burning of sugar for fuel happens in the body when most of our calories consumed are from carbohydrates—no need to waste any thought on this. The simple recipes and whole foods in your upcoming Challenge are packed with micronutrients and some fiber.

More things we can ignore that make diets *too hard*

Calorie counting and calorie restriction, counting points of any kind, portion control, protein and fat restriction, salt restriction, obsessing over the number on a scale, and even endless cardio sessions. *You are welcome!*

Effective weight loss is MOSTLY diet driven. Workout habits are healthy to stack with your diet, but it does not have the impact on fat loss that your diet will. Exercise is excellent for our healthy lifestyle. When you do add activity to your weekly routines, please don't go to extremes with this. Too much of anything can be a negative… even too much of a "good thing." You don't need to overdo your workouts, and I would argue that you shouldn't for optimal health. Yes, go hard (*80 percent of your max capacity*) for a minimum amount of time to get the best results—*the minimum effective dose.* For example, I advise my clients to do timed three-minute high-intensity intervals of *anything* for three sets, with one minute of rest between them to get their heart rate up and break a good sweat. Under fifteen minutes is all you need for great results. This workout can be achieved with a rowing machine, a bike, or bodyweight exercises (no equipment at all). Less is more.

This is the concept of Hormesis—how a minor stressor is a positive, and too much of any stressor becomes a negative (see the graph below).

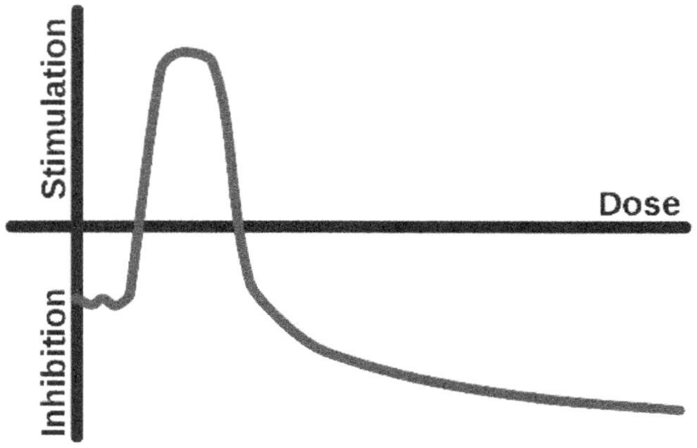

A little bit of stress (like exercise) is excellent for you (see stimulation), but too much can be harmful to you (see inhibition), just like any other stressor. People doing two hours of any cardio are often doing more harm than good to their bodies. Stresses in low doses are actually healthy for you. Training for and completing a marathon is super impressive for sure, but at what long-term cost to your health?

You don't need to work out at all during your 7 Day Challenge week to see and feel results that will give you positive momentum. You can continue to exercise if you were before your Challenge; no worries. If that is not part of your daily habits yet, consider adding it in after a couple of weeks of eating Keto, after you have effectively changed your fuel source from sugar to fat.

Bad info from "trusted sources"

Much of the bad information comes to us from sources we feel we know and trust. Many of these "trusted sources" are not motivated to admit when they made a mistake or are closed off from considering new information for various reasons. These trusted sources may choose to remain uninformed or to put out bad information due to a perceived lack of time, profit motivation, or they are just plain lazy. My bet is that it is all the above and more.

Even though the diet has been proven to be an effective tool for weight loss and has plenty of published studies to back those statements up, it still got ranked very low on the list. The U.S. News and World Report website lists the Keto Diet as twenty-one out of the twenty-four diets ranked in 2023. Many higher-ranking diets on their annual list are large corporate-owned, profit-driven companies selling prepackaged weight-loss meals. The knocks on the Keto Diet are not that it doesn't work but that it is restrictive and hard to sustain at times. From reading this book, you know I agree that the Keto Diet can be too complex, confusing, and even too challenging. My take here is, let's take something that works and make it simple. Win/win.

Many in the medical and nutritional consulting community still maintain that high-fat diets cause heart attacks and other diseases. This is an overgeneralized, incorrect statement, as many studies point to this not being true. The devil is in the details. The types of fats we consume do matter for our best health outcomes. There are healthy fats and less healthy fats. Not all fats are created equal. Avocadoes, salmon, and olive oil are just some super healthy fats. Unhealthy fats include margarine, fried foods, and processed snacks.

Our government leaders are still not advising anyone to eat this way even though eating the high-carb diet they have recommended for decades has led to 73.1% of our adult population being overweight, obese, or extremely obese (these rates are also published online by our government).

Who can we believe?!

Disclosure: I have a business degree, I'm a sales and marketing professional, and one of my goals is to earn profits in my business, too. So "trust me!" It would be hypocritical to think that just because I wrote a book or put a course together, I know what I'm talking about or could be deemed a trusted source. Please be skeptical, ask questions, and test things out for yourself!

Have strong opinions held loosely!

Be open to learning and testing things on yourself to prove if something will work for you (as you are doing here). There is no one-size-fits-all diet for all humans. Keto or anything else... Ultimately, whatever you are testing only matters if it works for YOU, not your neighbors, friends, relatives, or any random person posting their diet successes on social media.

One advantage I have in being trained as a professional marketer is I can spot marketing strategies that are at work to keep us fat and sick in the name of big company profits. If unaware and left to chance, we can easily succumb to what I like to call "Food Marketplace Manipulation (F.M.M.)." I'm revealing many of those tactics in this book.

Food Marketplace Manipulation

The 2020 Netflix docudrama *The Social Dilemma* focused on how big social media companies manipulate users with targeted algorithms that encourage addiction to their platforms. It also shows, fairly accurately, how platforms harvest personal data to target users with ads—and this has so far gone largely unregulated. The same is true with other profit-driven business sectors, including Big Food.

Big Food's Playbook for Profits:

✔ Food that is cheap to make and "cheap" for consumers to buy
✔ Food that is convenient
✔ Food that is "ready-made"
✔ Food that is "shelf stable"
✔ Food that is often full of salt and fat to make it hyper-palatable. Which can actually make us addicted to it
✔ Food with deceptive marketing and branding, such as "Low Fat," "All Natural," "Heart Healthy," and "Gluten Free"
✔ Food that's portable, manufacturer to trucks to stores and eventually, to table, does not matter how long it takes, as most foods by design are loaded with preservatives
✔ Food that is loaded with sugar or fake sugars; these

substances are addictive drugs—they drive repeat consumption

✔ Food that you can easily buy at gas stations, through windows, or vending machines

Big Food is motivated by profitable shareholder returns and not necessarily, if at all, by their customers' good health outcomes. If we keep buying Twinkies, they will keep selling us Twinkies. Do they even still make Twinkies?! I sure hope not... I just did a quick Amazon.com search. Yep, these things are still being sold to us. People are still buying them. My head and stomach hurt just thinking about the people eating Twinkies.

Not surprisingly, our environment impacts our decision-making process, and the tractor beam in the food marketplaces is strong! What and who makes up this F.M.M. camp? Food manufacturers, labeling practices, advertisements, government recommendations, drive-through menu boards, grocery store end cap displays, social media influencers, and many more.

We are being manipulated by marketplaces every day. We may not be aware of this, but we should start paying close attention to it. The food marketplace algorithm is always running, dictating what is being served up to us. The more we show an interest in X and ultimately, the more we buy of X, the more we are marketed X. It's like the TikTok algorithm in the grocery stores, serving us up more of what we are buying. It's all tracked to the penny. Since 73.1% percent of the U.S. adult population is currently overweight or obese, it's still serving up mostly highly processed, higher carbohydrate options. Sadly, not enough real, simple, healthy food. There are just not enough profits in real food. The profits are in the highly processed, carb-filled, fake foods.

For another example, let's look at the perfectly edited images of food and drinks on a Starbucks menu board. Take a look at the perfectly staged glass display case with the cake pops and other treats. That is some amazing and highly effective food and drink marketing going on there! The reason those foods and drinks make the cut on their beautiful signs or that space in the display case is that they have been proven to sell well! Those images/products are tested and tracked very closely to see how they perform in all markets. It's as simple as this... If we keep buying them, they will continue to feature and sell them to us. And *why wouldn't they?!* It's a winning business plan producing enormous profits for the company's shareholders. The good news is we have the power to change all of this based on our buying habits. If we hold out for more healthy options, companies will pivot to sell us those items, too. *We have the power in the end, and we vote with our dollars.* You see lots of "Keto" foods popping up in the food retailers. The large companies have realized they are starting to sell. The Challenge is that "Keto" labeling does not always equal healthy or even real food.

We have been unknowingly voting for highly processed carbs for many decades with our spending habits. With the Starbucks sign example, there are very few food and drink options that fall into a low-carb, Keto Diet outline. If your goal is to eat Keto, you must be intentional when ordering at Starbucks to bypass the other 19,000-plus options. Starbucks shareholders do not care if you are Keto or not! Now, we can and will make the food markets work for us, but we must be aware of all the traps in the marketplace.

I'm not just picking on Starbucks... in fact, I love their zero-carb green teas and low-carb sous vide egg bites, too. Their zero-carb Pike's Place black coffee is certainly drinkable. I love how their baristas are trained to ask for our name and put it on this fancy cup for you. People love it when their names are used! Everyone's favorite word is their own name. I love Starbucks AND am hyper-aware of this "food dilemma." I am very intentional about what I order when I am out in the food marketplaces to eat according to my goals. I'm taking control of eating to ensure it is on MY purpose!

The food market is not making eating Keto easy. Keto foods may not be advertised as "Hot 'n' Ready" in today's food marketplace, but they are there if you know what to look for. They come in the form of real, whole foods, like meats, cheeses, and some low-carb vegetables and fruits.

More food market manipulation from places you would least expect (like our government).

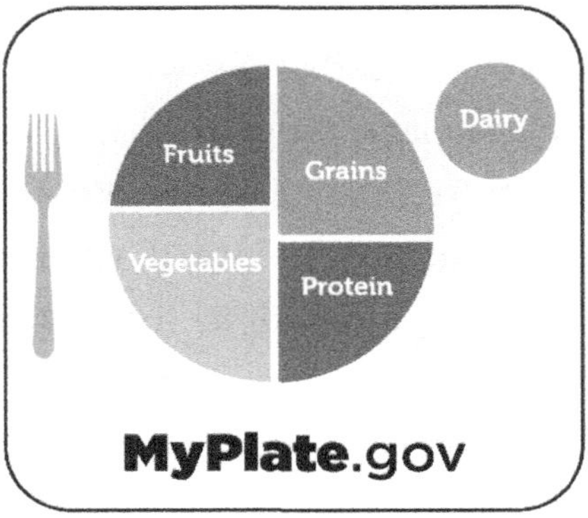

At www.myplate.gov, you can see this visual outline of a plate for eating healthily, published first in 2009 and still there today. These recommendations include plenty of high-carb starchy vegetables, high-carb fruits, and whole-grain foods. There is no mention of counting carbohydrates or limiting them at all. If following these recommendations, it's easy to see no one will be burning fat for fuel anytime soon. There is no mention of the importance of healthy fat consumption; rather, they point out to move to low-fat or even fat-free dairy. *Sigh... fat is not the enemy, it's sugar (processed carbs).*

Yes, these guidelines will ensure you will be burning sugar for fuel all the time. These guidelines will further ensure you have food cravings every couple of hours, as your insulin spikes after each high-carb meal and then comes crashing down again. You will never be directing your body to use fat for fuel. Maybe we should try doing the opposite of what brought 73.1% percent of the U.S. adult population to becoming overweight and obese?!

What do we have to lose? Well... a whole lot of belly fat and a bunch of diseases. These eating guidelines are woefully outdated and flat-out egregious!

Egregious

1. Outstandingly bad; shocking.

Synonyms: appalling, horrific, horrifying, awful, dreadful, ghastly, hideous, horrendous, atrocious, outrageous, monstrous, nightmarish, heinous, dire, unspeakable, shameful, flagrant, glaring, blatant, scandalous, unforgivable, intolerable.

Congratulations, you are taking charge here with testing Keto for yourself easily and effectively! Unfortunately, this bad information is leading to *bad inflammation* in our bodies! It's time to be accountable for our own health and to fact-check everything. We must be our own advocates and test things out for ourselves to see what works for us and what does not. Be proactive and intentional when you assemble the team that will support your health and happiness goals.

Keto convenience foods—paying for convenience, *but at what cost to our health?*

I also recommend avoiding most "Keto" processed, packaged food. Those usually contain low-carb, alternative sweeteners that taste like sugar. It's a slippery slope with the sweet ingredients companies use to make the foods taste like the sugar-laden products we are all addicted to. As such, these sugar alternatives might send you on a relapse back to binge eating more unhealthy foods.

Everything with low-carb counts is marketed with "Keto" or "Keto approved" on the packaging to appeal to the growing number of low-carb shoppers. It's a marketing strategy that works. This is a similar marketing tactic used to appeal to people trying to avoid grains as they want to be gluten-free. Big Food companies will produce more processed, high-carb, unhealthy foods with no grain and label them gluten-free to sound healthier. Yes, no gluten, but the ten other ingredients you can't pronounce may be worse for you than the gluten.

I love convenience, and who doesn't? That's why buying these boxed keto products with all the processed ingredients is so tempting. You can still get convenience and keep it healthy low carb with tasty, real foods.

You have all that in this 7 Day Challenge all set to go for you!

2

TOO MANY DAILY DECISIONS WITH OUR FOOD AND DRINK

Decisions, decisions, decisions...

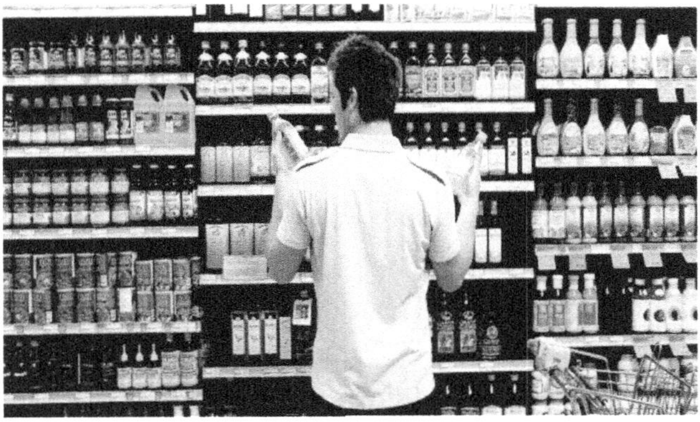

Decisions are the enemy of willpower

It's been proven that after seventy-five conscious decisions (about the number involved in one unplanned grocery store shopping trip), you will have exhausted your daily limit of willpower. So just by making hundreds of everyday food and drink decisions alone, we will run out of this valuable limited willpower every day at some point, sooner rather than later. Then we become vulnerable to bad decisions, including what we eat and drink.

So many food decisions are made on mindless autopilot

Is it your fault that you are overweight, obese, or extremely obese? Not entirely. You have been doing the best you can with the information that you have, right? In the past, when you ate too many carbs, you were constantly battling hunger pangs and had out-of-control food cravings. I found it eye-opening that studies show we all have a willpower limit daily. Knowing this, we don't need to feel bad about it... it's a thing that happens to everyone. Awareness of this fact is vital, so you can leverage what willpower you do have to work in your favor! After *digesting* the information in this course, you will have no more excuses! You will have the key information, and you will have an action plan!

The daily food dilemma...

What am I going to eat today?

How many food-based decisions do we make in a day? More than you may realize...

One study out of Cornell asked people this very question. On average, participants in the study guessed they would make about **14** food and drink-based decisions per day. When the participant's decisions were carefully tracked over time, the average daily number was a whopping **227.**

Almost all diets work for weight loss. Yep, for a limited time... as long as you stay on them. When you don't have a plan for eating, it's easy to run through your willpower and start struggling. A heavy overall decision day will lead to your willpower running out and your quality of decisions dropping earlier that day. As you realize, we make many more decisions outside of what we will eat and drink on any given day. Eating and drinking decisions alone put us over the threshold if we don't have a plan. By eliminating our daily eating decisions with a simple system, we support our willpower supply for better decision-making on everything!

Definition of willpower

☞ The ability to delay gratification and resist short-term temptations to meet long-term goals
☞ The capacity to override an unwanted thought, feeling, or impulse
☞ The conscious, effortful regulation of the self by the self
☞ A limited resource capable of being depleted

Willpower impacts every area of our lives

We rely on our supply of willpower to exercise, diet, save money, quit smoking, stop drinking, overcome procrastination, and ultimately, accomplish any of our goals in life.

Roy F. Baumeister, a social psychologist at Florida State University and author of the book, *Willpower: Rediscovering the Greatest Human Strength*, argues that willpower plays a part in all our decisions and that willpower fluctuates. When asked to name their greatest strengths, they often cite honesty, kindness, humor, courage, or other virtues. Surprisingly, self-control or willpower came in dead last among virtues studied in research with over one million people. The most successful people, Baumeister contends, don't have super-strong willpower when making decisions. Instead, they conserve their willpower by developing *habits and routines* to reduce stress in their lives. He says these people use their self-control or willpower not to get through crises but to avoid them. By design, they make important decisions early in the day and early in the week before decision fatigue sets in. Your Challenge outline for eating Keto is supporting your early strategic decisions!

Decision fatigue

This is the deteriorating quality of decisions made by an individual after a lengthy decision-making session during a given day. It leaves the person in a depleted state and hence, less likely to exert self-control effectively. This breakdown in the decision-making process is terrible news for any hope of dieting success. It's easy to make bad decisions in today's manipulative food marketplaces if you don't have a plan.

Lack of willpower is the greatest obstacle to change, and decisions themselves reduce this limited supply of willpower. We make thousands of decisions daily without even being aware of the number. Therefore, dieting, a daily series of food and drink-based decisions, would have a low success rate. *Our willpower runs out daily.* If we rely on willpower alone for success, we are indeed doomed to have our diets or anything else in our lives fail. Studies suggest that we make 35,000 decisions per day all in. It's no wonder we are mentally exhausted at the end of any day.

Consider that the diversity of product selection has expanded exponentially over the years. The average American supermarket in 1976 carried 9,000 different SKUs, whereas fifteen years later, that figure ballooned to 30,000. It is estimated that there are currently one million SKUs in the U.S., and the average supermarket carries 40,000 of them. The coffee shop chain Starbucks boasted in 2003 that it offered each customer 19,000 "beverage possibilities" at every store, and that was before their new "superheated" option, which multiplied the number even further.

The higher the *quantity* of daily decisions, the lower the *quality* of our daily decisions.

Think of eating the wrong kind of food later in the day as the proof... most likely, right before bed, the worst time to be eating. Eating right before bed leads to disrupted sleep as your body digests food when it should be doing other things. Fatigue leads to hormone disruption, which leads to feeling hungrier the next day. This often becomes a vicious cycle that wreaks havoc on your health and weight loss efforts.

You may be asking yourself, "How the hell do I get anything else done in my life with this many daily decisions?" That's a fair question. I would ask, "What if you were given back those two hundred and twenty-seven daily decisions?" The possibilities are endless for you with your newfound free time and your extra brain capacity. With your Challenge eating outline, I am giving you back these food and drink decisions every day. What will you do with all that extra willpower in your day? *I can't wait to see, as the possibilities are endless!*

Q: "How do I make discipline and willpower automatic"?
A: "A simple system that removes all decisions."

We gave you the answer to this very important question with this Challenge. In this 7 Day Air Fryer Challenge we are going to take thousands of weekly decisions all the way down to zero. Fewer decisions are needed, less decision fatigue, and more willpower for you to start this coming week!

With a system for your diet (this Challenge outline), your weekly eating decisions go from 1,589 to zero.

3

OUR FUEL SOURCE IS WRONG

Fuel source matters

When you are struggling with cravings and feel hungry all the time, your diet is doomed to fail sooner rather than later. Not only that, but these cravings and hunger pains make your diet and life inefficient. How does anyone stay on task if they always obsess about food and need to eat every three hours?

What happens when I eat 200 to 300 Grams of carbohydrates per day, every day of the week? For many, it's a recipe for disaster. When people eat food containing carbohydrates, their digestive system breaks down the digestible carbs into sugar, which enters the bloodstream. As blood sugar levels rise, the pancreas produces insulin, a hormone that prompts cells to absorb blood sugar for energy use now or to store it for later. This "stored for later" sugar becomes fat in the worst places and then hangs around for a long time in your body. Sugar is a dirty fuel, and it's just not optimal for most of us.

What happens when I eat fat while at the same time limiting my carbohydrate intake? Ketone bodies are made in the liver from the breakdown of fats from your food or from fat stores in your body. Ketone bodies are formed when there is insufficient sugar to supply the body's fuel needs. This process is a positive for weight loss as this process will cause you to lose body fat, that dreaded "stored for later" fat that is so hard to lose.

Change is hard

It's made even more challenging when many of our "trusted sources" still recommend this low-grade fuel source as a way to stay healthy and lose weight. This proven path to illness is known as the Standard American Diet. It's time for a radical change from the S.A.D. to something completely different if we expect to see a change in our body composition for the better. Again, what do we have to lose? *How about stubborn belly fat and disease?*

Changing our body's fuel source - *made simple.*

Sugar Burning Mode > Carbs, when daily consumption is *unlimited*, allow the body to burn sugar for fuel.

Fat Burning Mode > Carbs, when daily consumption is *limited*, direct the body to burn fat for fuel.

Pretty simple, right? Rather than relying on counting calories, limiting portion sizes, and resorting to extreme cardio workouts, this low-carb lifestyle takes an entirely different approach to weight loss and upgrading your health. Different is good, trust me! It can work in part because it changes the very fuel source that your body uses to stay energized... from burning sugar to burning fat for its main fuel source. Sometimes you need radical change to experience radical (aka good) results.

Reminder: You always need consistent actions to get any kind of result.

Fat and protein make us feel full

Hungry still? Fat and protein are levers to pull based on how full you feel. Eating more fat or protein is the answer if you are hungry. Consuming less dietary fat will direct your body to burn your body fat for fuel. Consuming more fat from your food, your body will burn this first, and your weight loss may slow a bit. Depending on your unique situation, that may be just fine. Feeling full contributes to sustaining this way of eating, and we know that makes it a lifestyle, not a diet. You never want to feel like you are starving to death or to struggle with food cravings if you hope to sustain any eating outline. Once you get days into your Challenge, you will notice you are not as consumed with these feelings anymore! That's a sign you are on the right track!

Sugar is an addictive street drug

Why am I starving all the time? Most of us are unknowingly doing addictive drugs every day. We are mainlining a dangerous drug that goes by the street name *sugar.* This drug has been overdosed on in the typical Standard American Diet for decades and is responsible for countless diseases and deaths.

The default Standard American Diet consists of eating and then burning 200 to 300 Grams of highly processed carbohydrates (or sugar) for fuel per day. The vicious cycle of consuming sugar as our primary fuel source causes ravenous food cravings, wild mood swings, and always feeling like you're starving to death, even after eating your last meal only a few hours ago.

A highly cited study in the journal *Neuroscience & Biobehavioral Reviews* found that sugar, as pervasive as it is, meets the criteria for a substance of abuse and may be addictive to those who binge on it. It does this by affecting the chemistry of the limbic system, the part of the brain associated with emotional control. The study found that intermittent access to sugar can lead to behavioral and neurochemical changes resembling the effects of an abused substance. There is a large dopamine hit to the brain when sugar is consumed, which makes us crave it even more.

How consuming sugar causes hunger and cravings

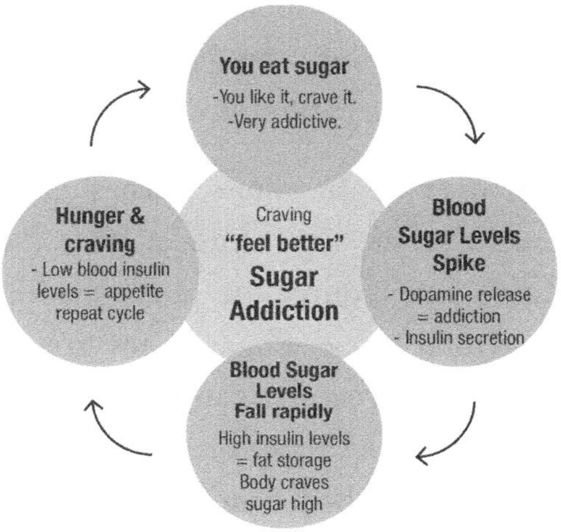

I know I have had issues with sugar, and I still do when I have chosen to consume it for any reason. I know this because I notice I can't control my consumption once I get into this sugar addiction craving cycle again. Sounds a lot like any other drug addiction, right? One bite of an offending sugar-laced food can trigger me. One potato chip soon becomes the entire bag. If you deep fry sugar in processed oils, it's even worse. It's all or nothing most of the time with sugar consumption. Not taking the first bite takes less discipline than trying to stop after just one or two bites. Stopping once the addiction cycle has started is almost impossible. It's the nature of a sugar drug fix.

It's important to note that any carbohydrates get converted to sugar in the body. Our bodies are doing a lot of work to deal with this sugar, so it makes sense it would make you tired in the process. From pizza to apples to cane sugar, it's a roller coaster ride that spike insulin levels after eating carbohydrates and then crashes hard shortly after that. When energy crashes, we become hungry again, not to mention we feel wiped out. This cycle of ups and downs every few hours a day translates into many diseases in the body, including obesity.

Many unhealthy, overweight adults burn sugar for their fuel source 100 percent of the time, forever. It is the easy, cheap, default alternative fuel source in most marketplaces when looking for something to eat. Sugar tastes great, and in many internal aisles in your grocery store, it comes loaded with enough added preservatives to sit on the shelf for months, and even years, without going bad. Since people get addicted to it, you have repeat consumption, which means more sales. It's Big Food's wet dream for more profits.

We all kinda knew that consuming straight sugar like a Pixie Stick is not good for us, right? We certainly realize that it's not really healthy to grab your spoon and dip it into the "all-natural" bag of cane sugar for an everyday snack. The liquid version in energy drinks and soda is an even easier path to getting sugar into the body and brain. It's easy to overdose on this liquid form of sugar, making it a huge problem.

The next less obvious, but no less bad for you, foods are the packaged products with ingredients you can't even pronounce sitting on the shelves of the grocery stores. Here, we need to carefully read the labels to see how many carbs we are looking at in each serving and what other nasty ingredients are in the so-called "food." We must be on guard with misleading food labels like "gluten-free" or "heart healthy." These packaging labels sure sound healthy, but be sure to look at the whole picture via the ingredients label. *Buyer beware!*

It's this next tier of foods that trip most of us up when we are looking to lose fat and regain our health. Where many people don't connect the dots is on the other real foods, like certain fruits, starchy vegetables, and whole grains. Many of these foods are packed with carbohydrates that, if over-consumed, will not allow your body to burn fat for fuel, either. Here, we must be aware of our daily carb counts if our goal is to eat Keto and burn fat for our primary fuel source.

We can include some low-carb fruits and vegetables in our keto lifestyle in moderation, as there are some good micronutrients and fiber in these foods that are good for us. I've done the carb limiting for you in your Challenge, so this will be smooth sailing for your Challenge week!

Red Flags that our fuel source is wrong:

- The fact that you are "starving to death" every three hours of every day.
- The fact that you can't stop consuming large quantities of this type of food once you start eating it.
- The fact that you suffer from energy crashes every couple of hours, all day long, every day.
- The fact that the majority of the U.S. adult population is overweight, obese, and extremely obese.
- The fact that the majority of the U.S. adult population is sick (obesity is a disease).

This fifty-plus-year "S.A.D. experiment" has proven to us in the U.S. that consuming heavily processed carbs is causing illnesses of all kinds, including obesity. We are doing that here! It's way past time to try something different, but thankfully, it's not too late.

Okay, what else actually matters?!

Fuel source frequency matters

My definition of *dieting insanity*: Eating six or more meals and snacks per day and always being hungry.

"Optional" eating is *optimal.* I prefer the flexibility of when I choose to eat to be "optional". With fat as your fuel source, you can go longer between meals comfortably without the stress of hunger pangs or any cravings. With sugar as your fuel source, it's painful to go longer than a couple of hours without feeling like you are starving. With fat as your fuel source, your biology will no longer dictate your mealtimes. It's very liberating. You can eat *on purpose* by taking control of your fuel source.

As I edit this part of Reason #3 that diets don't work, it's 1:18 p.m. on a Tuesday. After waking up, I consumed a "Keto Coffee" and a second black cup around noon today. No solid food yet... Eating solid food feels optional to me. I usually eat two meals a day (usually made in my air fryer). Sometimes by design, I'll eat three meals in a day if I'm doing something social with friends or family that involves a meal. Eating truly becomes optional when you don't have cravings all the time. You don't have to always be obsessing about and then digesting food all day long.

It's a more even-burning fuel source when you start burning fat for fuel instead of sugar.

Fuel source quality matters

Examples of quality sourced food on the labels: ***wild caught, organic, pasture raised, grass fed/grass finished***

We should all pay attention to how our food is sourced, whether we are eating Keto or not. Now, I don't recommend obsessing over this, but make healthy choices when you can. I know some feel they can't afford to eat the higher quality sourced foods. Actually, it's very affordable to eat high quality sourced food while living a keto lifestyle. When investing in yourself as you are doing with this Challenge, your health return on investment is enormous when choosing to buy quality sourced, whole foods. It's money well invested if you are spending it on quality sourced food.

Fuel source micronutrients matter

We are making it a goal to increase our health and happiness, and that is directly affected by the vitamins and minerals we consume through the foods we choose to eat every day. By design, I added very nutrient-dense foods to heat and eat with your 7 Day Air fryer Challenge. You will notice that I prioritized animal-sourced foods for these simple recipes in your challenge. Consuming animal-sourced foods is the most efficient way for our bodies to get and digest more of these healthy micronutrients. You can eat Keto and get your daily nutrients from a strictly plant-based diet, but it is more challenging and takes way more careful planning to cover all your micronutrient bases. To look and feel your best, it will require you to consume some extra supplements, too. If you prefer vegetables, you can take the outline in this Challenge and adjust it to your preferences to include low-carb veggies or anything else more to your liking. You will have the concepts and the simple system, just swap out the foods staying under the carb limit, and you are good to go.

"When in doubt, eat more steak!"

Keeping it simple! A piece of steak with some grass-fed Kerrygold butter on top is one example of a complete, healthy Keto meal. Here are the micronutrients in this simple yet delicious Keto meal:

Ribeye Steak:

Vitamins: A, B1, B2, B3, B5, B6, B9, B12, D, E, K, plus Choline and CoQ10.
Minerals: Calcium, Chromium, Cobalt, Copper, Iron, Magnesium, Manganese, Molybdenum, Phosphorous, Potassium, Selenium, Sodium, Zinc.

Grass fed Kerrygold butter:

Vitamins: A, B1, B2, B3, B5, B7, B9, B12, D, E, K, plus Choline and CoQ10.
Minerals: Calcium, Chromium, Cobalt, Copper, Iodine, Iron, Magnesium, Manganese, Molybdenum, Phosphorous, Potassium, Selenium, Sodium, Zinc.

The incredible, edible egg

Aren't all eggs the same!? Not even close... I will gladly invest $6.99 in a dozen free-range, organic, "pastured" eggs at the local grocery store. What a value! I opt for these quality sourced eggs produced by happy, well-cared-for chickens that frolic freely in the fresh air and sunshine as they graze on pastures of nutrient-dense grass and bugs. I don't want to eat grass or bugs directly, so I am fine with these healthy chickens doing that for me, as it then translates into higher micronutrients for you and me when we enjoy their eggs. If you buy the above eggs and then spend less on some eggs that came from a sad environment of poorly fed, overcrowded, antibiotic-filled hens and crack them open side-by-side, you will see a huge difference in the color of the yolks. The eggs from the pasture-raised, well-cared-for hens are a dark yellow, and the other will look pale. As you will see below, the dark yellow yolks are full of more nutrients.

"Happy hens have more vitamin D!"

In comparison to a conventional egg, pasture-raised eggs contain:

- ☑ **1/3 less cholesterol**
- ☑ **1/4 less saturated fat**
- ☑ **2/3 more Vitamin A**
- ☑ **2 times more omega-3 fatty acids**
- ☑ **3 times more Vitamin E**
- ☑ **7 times more beta carotene**
- ☑ **6 times more Vitamin D**

In 2008, a follow-up study showed that the significant sunlight exposure the hens enjoy translates from the sun to the hens to the eggs in the form of increased levels of Vitamin D—*by as much as four to six times more than conventional eggs!* Those other eggs might be on sale for $0.99/dozen, but at what cost to your health?! Not suitable for the chickens and not good for us. Eggs are a staple in my keto lifestyle, and I include them in your challenge, too. *It pays to invest more to get quality eggs!*

"Clean" versus "dirty" Keto matters

Clean Keto: Nutrient-dense foods, wild-caught, grass-fed, pasture-raised, and organic food ingredients when your budget allows (it's really not that expensive if you shop with a plan). Remember, the cost of being obese far *outweighs* the cost of organic or grass-fed food purchases over time. I have found I throw less food away, too. Fresh vegetables and fruits can go bad quickly, and then you have to toss them out.

Dirty Keto: Low-nutrient foods are made up of lower carbs, but unhealthy ingredients are included, too. Examples of these would include foods made with highly processed, inflammation-causing seed oils like soy, corn, and canola. Farm-raised fish, commercially raised eggs, and artificially sweetened foods as well. Not all Keto foods are created equal for health... In fact, when any food is "created," be aware of what is in it, even if it is marketed as "Keto-friendly." Just because something is "Keto" does not guarantee it's healthy for you to eat a lot of. Some of these highly processed "Keto foods" that I see in the market are not healthy at all. These packaged foods are okay occasionally but don't make them a staple in your weekly meal planning. They can be "trigger foods," causing you to crave the high-carb versions of these foods.

Ketosis, a power tool for fat loss and many other health benefits.

The state in the body known as ketosis is where Keto gets its name from. Ketosis happens when you go for a period of time limiting your carb intake (usually to under 50 grams a day), for as little as a few days. Lots of beneficial things happen when you are in a state of ketosis, not the least of which is: you will start to lose visceral fat (fat around your organs), and over time this can cause your pants to fall down. Great problems to have! Once in ketosis, your hunger and cravings will diminish. Your body will begin burning fat for fuel instead of sugar, and you will begin to see and feel positive changes. This is known as keto momentum. Following a Ketogenic Diet is the most efficient approach that results in nutritional ketosis. I make it easy to follow Keto here.

Once you have gotten into the state of ketosis by limiting your carb intake, you should begin to notice these benefits that will make losing fat way less painful than with many other diets.

- ➤ Less hunger promotes easier periods of fasting
- ➤ Being less hungry promotes being in a caloric deficit
- ➤ Reduction of hunger cravings

When I talk about making willpower automatic, the above benefits go a long way to supporting your success. When you are not starving all the time and don't have uncontrollable cravings, you will have an easier time sustaining this way of eating as you lose fat along the way.

Here are some of the key benefits for the body and brain of getting into ketosis, supported by published studies:

Weight loss

One of the most well-known benefits of the Keto Diet is its potential for weight loss. By limiting your carbohydrates, the body is forced to burn stored fat for energy, leading to weight loss.

Blood sugar regulation

The Keto Diet may also be beneficial for individuals with type 2 diabetes or insulin resistance, as it can improve blood sugar control and reduce insulin resistance.

Brain function

The brain can also benefit from being in ketosis, as ketones are a more efficient fuel source for the brain than glucose. Studies have shown that ketones can improve cognitive function, reduce inflammation in the brain, and even have potential therapeutic effects for neurological conditions such as epilepsy and Alzheimer's disease.

Reduced inflammation

The Keto Diet has been shown to reduce inflammation in the body, which is a contributing factor to many chronic diseases such as heart disease and cancer.

Improved heart health

The Keto Diet may also have benefits for heart health, as it has been shown to reduce levels of triglycerides (a type of fat in the blood) and increase levels of HDL cholesterol (the "good" cholesterol).

Seven days is not enough time to realize all the potential long-term benefits of the Keto Diet; you need to make this a lifestyle. A week is just enough time for you to see and feel the potential of this becoming a lifestyle for you. Most people will start burning fat for fuel and be in the state of ketosis in just seven days. Once you have this 7 Day Challenge system in place, you can easily rinse and repeat as long as you want. You can choose to swap out other low-carb recipes according to your unique tastes, too.

Recruiting your hormones to work *for you*

When you systematically limit your daily carb consumption in as little as seven days, most people will dip into this fat-burning state of ketosis. When you do, you automatically reset your hunger hormone, ghrelin. This change results in fewer cravings and feelings of hunger, which supports making this way of eating sustainable. Inviting our hormones to work for us is a welcome change instead of constantly fighting against us.

> Following diet-induced weight loss, the circulating concentrations of several hormones and nutrients influencing appetite were altered when participants were ketotic (*in ketosis*), compared with after refeeding. **The study proves: .48 mmol/L to reduce ghrelin and to reduce subjective appetite.**

Other activities that accelerate ketosis, along with limiting your daily carb intake:

Intermittent fasting

Intermittent fasting is a pattern of eating where you cycle between periods of fasting and eating. One of the benefits of intermittent fasting is that it can help the body get into ketosis more quickly.

Exercise

Exercise is another way to promote ketosis, as it can increase the body's demand for energy and help burn through stored glucose.

Medium-chain triglycerides (MCTs)

MCTs are a type of fat that can be rapidly metabolized into ketones by the liver. Consuming MCT oil or adding MCTs into your diet can help increase ketone production and promote ketosis.

Exogenous ketones

As the name suggests, it is getting ketones from outside the body. Exogenous ketones are ketones that are consumed in supplement form. They can help increase levels of ketones in the blood and promote ketosis, even in individuals who are not following a Keto Diet.

MCT oil is a healthy fat game changer!

Medium-chain triglyceride (MCT) oil is a popular dietary supplement widely used for its potential health benefits. MCT oil is a type of fat that is distilled down from coconut or palm kernel oil, and it is composed of fatty acids with shorter chain lengths than those found in most other dietary fats.

Health benefits of consuming MCT oil:

Weight loss and weight management

In several studies, MCT oil has been shown to help with weight loss and weight management. One study published in the *American Journal of Clinical Nutrition* found that consuming MCT oil as part of a weight loss diet led to greater weight loss and fat loss than consuming olive oil. Another study published in the *Journal of Nutrition* found that consuming MCT oil as part of a weight maintenance diet led to more significant weight loss and fat loss over a six-month period compared to consuming olive oil. These findings suggest that MCT oil may be a helpful tool for those looking to manage their weight.

Improved cognitive function

In some studies, MCT oil has been shown to positively affect cognitive function. One study published in the *Journal of Alzheimer's Disease* found that consuming MCT oil improved cognitive function in people with mild cognitive impairment. Another study published in *Nutritional Neuroscience* found that consuming MCT oil improved cognitive function in healthy adults. These findings suggest that MCT oil may be useful for improving cognitive function in healthy individuals and those with cognitive impairment.

Increased energy and endurance

MCT oil has been shown to increase energy and endurance in some studies. One study published in the *Journal of Nutritional Science and Vitaminology* found that consuming MCT oil before exercise increased endurance and improved performance in endurance athletes. Another study published in the *Journal of the Academy of Nutrition and Dietetics* found that consuming MCT oil before exercise led to increased energy expenditure and improved exercise performance in overweight men. These findings suggest that MCT oil may be a useful tool for improving energy and endurance during exercise.

Improved digestion and gut health

In some studies, MCT oil has been shown to positively affect digestion and gut health. One study published in the *Journal of Gastroenterology* found that consuming MCT oil improved digestion and reduced symptoms of irritable bowel syndrome (I.B.S.) in people with I.B.S. Another study published in the journal *Digestion* found that consuming MCT oil improved symptoms of diarrhea and bloating in people with mild gastrointestinal disorders. These findings suggest that MCT oil may be a useful tool for improving digestion and gut health in people with digestive disorders.

In this Challenge we are adding this MCT oil to our coffee, tea, and any of our foods (even drizzling on top of foods). MCT oil is an incredible tool for pushing your body into ketosis and making you feel full as well. It's 14 grams of healthy fat per tablespoon. This highly distilled MCT oil is tasteless, so it will not impact the flavor of your food or drinks. You can add 1 tablespoon to any drink, including water. I recommend starting with 1 tablespoon per day and building up from there to see how you feel.

Exogenous ketones, support for fat loss, and more

Exogenous ketones are supplements that contain beta-hydroxy-butyrate (B.H.B.), a type of ketone body that is produced by the liver during periods of fasting or carbohydrate restriction. Exogenous ketones can be consumed as a powder or a drink, designed to provide the body with an immediate source of ketones.

Health Benefits of Exogenous Ketones:

Weight Loss

Exogenous ketones may be helpful for those looking to lose weight by reducing their caloric intake. One of the most commonly cited benefits of exogenous ketones is their ability to aid in weight loss. A study published in the journal *Obesity* in 2018 found that consuming exogenous ketones as a supplement increased the levels of ketones in the blood and resulted in a decrease in appetite and food intake.

Athletic Performance

Exogenous ketones have also been studied for their potential to improve athletic performance. A study published in the *Journal of Physiology* in 2016 found that consuming exogenous ketones as a supplement improved endurance performance in trained cyclists. The researchers suggested that this may be due to the ability of ketones to provide an alternative energy source during prolonged exercise.

Brain Function

A study published in the journal *Neurobiology of Aging* in 2016 found that consuming exogenous ketones as a supplement improved cognitive function in patients with mild cognitive impairment. The researchers suggested that this may be due to the ability of ketones to improve cerebral blood flow and provide an alternative energy source for the brain. Ketones have also been shown to have neuroprotective effects and may benefit brain function.

Diabetes

Exogenous ketones may also be beneficial for those with diabetes. A study published in the journal *Diabetes* in 2017 found that consuming exogenous ketones as a supplement improved blood glucose control in patients with type 2 diabetes. The researchers suggested that this may be due to the ability of ketones to increase insulin sensitivity and improve glucose uptake in the muscles.

How do I know if I am in ketosis?

I debated if I should include this topic in my book on how to do the simplest form of Keto ever. It's a bit "bio-hacky" as it involves a measuring device and a finger prick to obtain a droplet of blood to test for ketone levels. It is a visual, data-driven indicator that can motivate you as you start your Keto journey. It's totally optional, but I feel like some of you will want to do it, so I decided to include it here. *So here goes...*

We can measure ketone levels in our blood to see how we are doing from the digital display on a small, simple device. The state of ketosis is achieved when the level of ketone bodies accumulates in the bloodstream equal to or greater than .5 mmol/L.

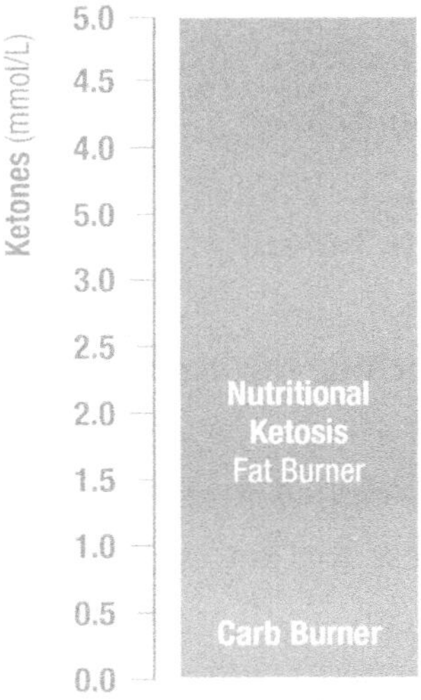

Your personal, real-time ketone data at your fingertips (literally).

The best way to tell whether you're in ketosis is to measure your ketone levels using a blood ketone measuring tool. If this sounds interesting to you, I recommend going to my online Challenge resource page to purchase the device and the testing strips. A link and Q.R. code in the references section at the end of this book take you right to these products to order them.

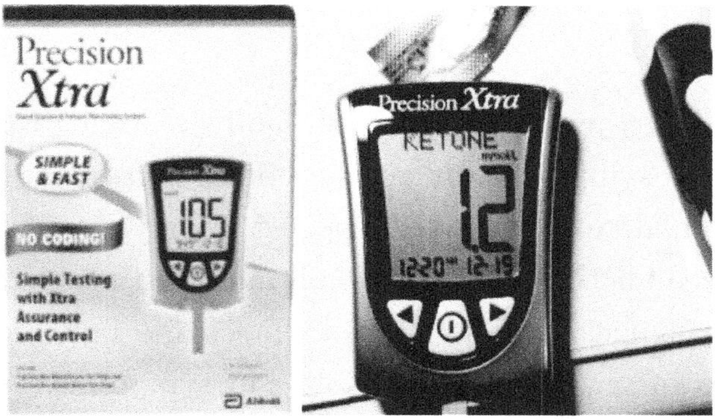

In addition to quantifying blood ketone levels with this little tool, there are several biological changes that your body may experience to help you identify a ketogenic state. These changes will be subjective and will vary by individual, as everyone is unique. These subjective feelings are things you will want to take note of to see if this is another benefit to you.

Getting into a ketogenic state can elicit euphoric effects, including:

- Increased energy
- Increased cognitive performance
- Mental clarity

Knowing your blood ketone levels can be powerful feedback and can be quite motivating. Don't worry about testing and tracking your blood ketone levels during your 7 Day Challenge first week. If you decide to rinse and repeat for a few months, it can be very beneficial to test/track your levels for a month or two.

Keto Flu

Overhauling the fuel source your body is used to can cause short-term symptoms for some people, known as the "Keto Flu." Again, detoxing is to be expected when you are getting off a drug as addictive as sugar. Going into the first few weeks of your Challenge, I recommend adding some targeted supplements to offset any possible Keto Flu symptoms. When you first start your Keto journey, you will lose some water weight, which can flush out some of your body's electrolyte stores, too. If you are not staying hydrated and adding some electrolyte supplements, you could feel bad as you transition in the short term. If you experience any annoying symptoms, they usually taper off a couple of weeks after changing your fuel source from sugar to fat. Not everyone will experience the effects of Keto Flu, but the following recommended actions will add additional support either way.

Recommendations to limit Keto Flu symptoms:

Drink plenty of water with electrolytes daily

Consume plenty of quality sea salt with your meals and in your water, too. A general rule of thumb on the amount of water is 90 ounces for women and 125 ounces for men per day. If you are working out and sweating, you may need to drink even more. I recommend Redmond's Sea Salt products to add to your water. It's good for you, and this quality sea salt has sixty-four minerals, too.

Consume exogenous ketone supplements daily

I recommend Real Ketones brand supplement as they include ketones and cover your important electrolytes, which contain magnesium and potassium. This brand is quality and less expensive than some other brands on the market. These supplements will help bridge the gap for you when changing your fuel source from sugar to fat, as we are doing in this Challenge.

Consume MCT oil daily

Data from a published study in 2018 showed that the healthy adults that were starting a Keto Diet, and consumed one teaspoon of MCT three times per day, produced more ketone bodies than the control group. In the same study, consuming one teaspoon of MCT three times per day improved the test group's mood and lowered the effects of the "Keto Flu."

4

SETTING GOALS BUT WITH NO VEHICLE FOR ACTION

If you go to the gym enough times, you become the type of person who is into fitness based on your actions. The beauty of this is we can change and upgrade our habits at any time. We can decide what type of people we want to become based on our actions via our habits. *Not* fake it till you make it... Do it till it becomes a habit! Goals are nothing... without actions!!

"Our habits are proof of the type of people we are."

With no system, no guarantees. Many of us set goals around dieting and many other things, but far fewer have a plan in place to ensure we take the actions to reach them. Some of us sustain an eating pattern with willpower alone for a time, but when willpower runs out, as it does, we then slip back into unhealthy habits, and frustration and depression follow soon after. You know the drill; we have all been there and gotten the XL-size T-shirts. Without a system for daily habits in place, the diet you were attempting to follow was just not sustainable for more than a short period of time.

Vision Boards and Goals

You need to *do* the thing, not just think about it. Have you seen or even completed a vision board before? Is that still even a thing? I actually put one such board together in 2020 to see if it could motivate me to reach my goals that year. I included the family, and we went nuts putting these boards together in the basement. It's a cool, creative, visual way to set some goals. It was a fun exercise, but it was still missing the key ingredient to making the goals happen... the boards don't account for the "how to" part.

Just like our goals, all the information in the world is useless if you don't take systematic actions to guarantee your results.

S.M.A.R.T. Goals?

This is an overused acronym in the business world for goal setting: ***S**pecific, **M**easurable, **A**ttainable, **R**elevant, and **T**ime-Bound.* But... it leaves out the crucial part... the "actions needed to accomplish" part. Goals alone, no matter how *smartly* they are constructed, guarantee neither actions nor results. In fact, forget goals. The concept of setting goals has been around forever. Goals themselves don't *do* anything. Goals are not actions. I have set many goals for all kinds of things over the years. It's an excellent framework to clarify a desired outcome, right? Set some goals... it's a concept that has been beaten to death in many published business how-to books, blog articles, podcasts, and T.E.D. Talks. Goals are a placeholder to provide a target, but they do not guarantee progress. Progress takes repeated action. *That is what we are doing here!*

"Goals without consistent action are missed... consistently."

How to win at *ANYTHING*

Why does the casino always win? They have a proven system... Of course, it's not just random luck that they continue to build enormous new casinos with an endless supply of their customers' gambling losses. Take for example, one of the casino's most popular card games, blackjack. Have you ever sat down or witnessed others sit down at a table in a casino to play blackjack with no training and no idea what they were doing? They don't know the game's rules, like when to take a hit or stay with the hand they have to give them the best chance to win. You could say they don't have a system. Some books and courses teach you all the "correct plays" based on statistical outcomes. These books teach the player a system to follow. Why? It removes the player's burden of having to make random decisions on each hand they are dealt. If the player sits long enough at a table, making too many decisions, they will end up losing money.

These soon-to-be huge losers are easy to spot in the casinos. They struggle to make decisions, as they have no knowledge of what they should do or frame of reference. They may start to go with hunches as the rest of the players roll their eyes and groan. These unskilled players may think their results are all based on luck! Trust me; it is lucky if they win for any length of time. They even rationalize that they are "due" for a particular card to come out of the deck next to give them a winning hand. They most likely have had some alcohol as well, to almost guarantee their decision-making is going from bad to worse. These players without a system will annoy everyone with a system at the table as they hold up the game, agonizing over every decision until their money is gone.

I trust you get the point I'm trying to sledgehammer home here. The casino has a proven system. Most players losing their money at the table do not. It's really that simple. The dealer never makes their own decisions on a hand. The decision is made for them based on a proven system of percentages for each and every hand. *Sound familiar?* Most dieters end up losing this way, too.

Awareness + Actions = Achievement

We now have an awareness from the information presented in this Challenge book about why we should do the thing. Now, how do we ensure that we will take action on it? We add a free tool, the calendar. Let's agree here that if we put something in our calendar, by definition, it's *non-negotiable, and we will do it no matter what.* We agree here to defend our calendar entries as though our health and happiness (and weight loss) depend on it because they do.

What decisions do we make every day, and what value do we give to each of them? Examples of high-priority decisions and goals might be: How we fuel our body, working out, reducing stress, sleep, what we are wearing, watching on streaming services, browsing on social media, spending time with kids, generating income, socializing with friends...

These non-negotiable priorities should include increasing your health and happiness, as defined by you. These top priorities for you should never be left to chance. These are the habits that are so important that it makes sense to reflect weekly on them. Whatever priorities make the cut for you, you will add them to your weekly calendar as non-negotiable appointments with yourself. These are the most important appointments for your week!

How we fuel our bodies is absolutely a non-negotiable priority for us! The number of days for your Challenge was not just a random number I pulled out of the air. We must plan how we fuel our bodies every week (thus, seven days).

Using your calendar to safeguard your success

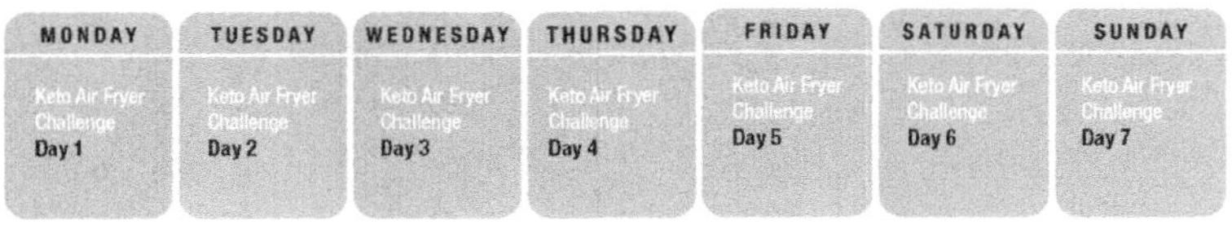
MONDAY
Keto Air Fryer Challenge Day 1
TUESDAY
Keto Air Fryer Challenge Day 2
WEDNESDAY
Keto Air Fryer Challenge Day 3
THURSDAY
Keto Air Fryer Challenge Day 4
FRIDAY
Keto Air Fryer Challenge Day 5
SATURDAY
Keto Air Fryer Challenge Day 6
SUNDAY
Keto Air Fryer Challenge Day 7

Calendar Entry = Non-Negotiable

➔ Use a free Google calendar with your free Gmail.com account (simply create one if you don't have one already).

7 Day Capsule Wardrobe System

"What am I going to wear today?"

We all spend too much time on decisions about what we are going to wear each day, too. Most of us tend to waste more time and brain energy on this daily decision than we should. Here is another example of a system highly effective people use so they can conserve their limited willpower. When you systematically organize your clothes by days in a week, this constitutes a *7 Day Capsule Wardrobe System.* This concept has been around forever because it works! This system for what you will wear also automatically reduces your daily decision fatigue around what to wear each day.

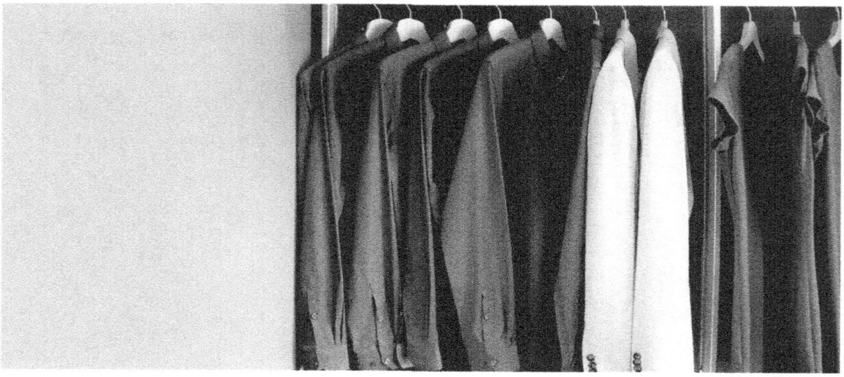

Many successful business people and celebrities have used this system for years to streamline productivity. I use it, too… a very accomplished person, like Albert Einstein, didn't want to waste his limited brainpower picking out an outfit every single morning. As we see in the history books, he had much better things to do!

Even some trendy thinking A-list celebrities today show us that having a system for a wardrobe can be hip. Lately, I am seeing a new term thrown around the internet called "outfit repeating." This sounds way hipper than a capsule wardrobe. Outfit repeating has become a celebrity badge of honor... *who knew?!* Kim Kardashian knows... She subscribes to wearing the same thing multiple times a week. Maybe I should have called my program "Simple Keto Meal Repeating" to sound more hip.

"Repetition is the mother of learning, the father of action, which makes it the architect of accomplishment."
—Zig Ziglar

High achievers like Steve Jobs, Mark Zuckerberg, Albert Einstein, and Kim Kardashian all have adopted this wardrobe system concept for the same reasons I laid out for you regarding our eating habits. Fewer decisions, more willpower, and added brain power to do other things.

I had unknowingly adopted this outfit-repeating concept in the last couple of years with my clothes. I noticed even though I would waste time looking over my entire closet every day (a massive waste of time and brain energy to start my day), I kept going back to the same shirt-pants-jacket-shoes combo over and over after wasting all that time. I was only wearing 20 percent of the clothes in my closet every week, no matter how long I stared at all the clothes every single day. And it was the same 20 percent.

I liked how I looked in a few select outfits, mostly color shades of black and blue and a lightweight material that felt good on my skin. I had sweaters that I never wore, as I didn't like the look or feel of them, yet they continued to take up space in my closet and brain for years. The fit of the few items I wore over and over was always flattering for my body type and therefore made me feel better when wearing them. *Look good, feel good.* My outfit repeating system was in place, giving me back even more time I had been wasting every day. As you might imagine, this practice increased my brain energy, too. Makes sense, right? Once I finally figured this out, I donated the rest of my unworn outfits to a local thrift store.

Now when shopping for clothes, which I rarely need to do anymore, I know exactly what to look for to match my personal brand, color, style, and fit. When I do find stuff I like, I will even buy pants or shirts in multiples if they have them in my size, as I struggle to find the right fit for me in most stores. You may not even realize you are doing it, but you also have your own predetermined criteria for your wardrobe. Trust me; you have a personal brand and a favorite look.

This week's wardrobe challenge for you:

Record what you wear for the next seven days (write it down). My bet is that you will see it's the same 20 percent of your wardrobe that you default to. You may even try on three or more outfits and all the combinations down to your shoes before, in the end… you go with that same 20 percent. Depleting your willpower with all these decisions before you even get out of the door is not a great way to start your day.

Take a look at your last six months of social media pictures and posts and any selfie shots in your phone's picture gallery app. The fit, the colors, the style, the material… If you are like me, I bet it's the same type of look. It's the look that makes you look and feel your best! It's your signature look! I bet at least half of the clothes in your closet have not been worn in over months or more. With this system in place, you will now have zero wardrobe decisions to make, and you will look and feel great every day. Can it really be this simple? Yes! Do this wardrobe challenge, and then you can donate the rest of your unworn items to a local thrift store.

7 Day Capsule Meal System, ***a system for eating on purpose***

Is there a "1 size fits all" dietary outline for every human? **No.**

Is there a "1 size fits all" system to ensure you eat a certain way? **Yes!**

Use This 7 Day Keto Diet Air Fryer Challenge outline to guarantee your willpower and success at eating Keto. I have included a variety of base Keto staple foods (like a wardrobe with basic combinations). We are talking savory salmon and ribeye steaks here, not skinny jeans and sweatshirts! The beauty of any system is that once you put the framework in place, you can always add/delete, rinse, and repeat. You can always customize the system to fit your unique tastes.

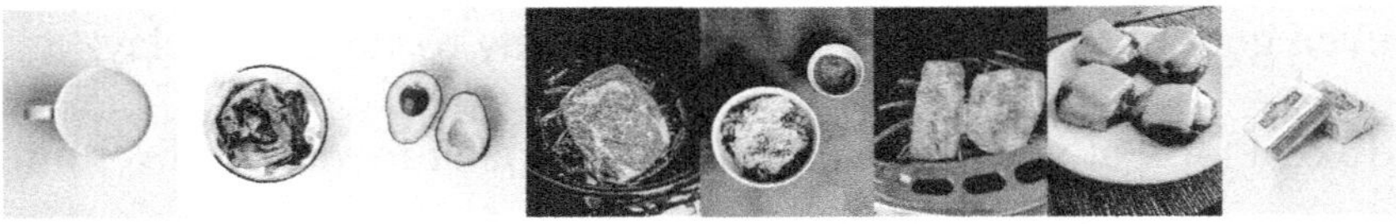

To be an effective eater, you must have an organized outline of foods to shop for and prepare for the week. It's predetermined. No decisions around food equal less decision fatigue overall for your day, which conserves your willpower. *Nothing this important should ever be left to chance!* By planning seven days out, we are eliminating all of our daily brain-zapping food and drink decisions. As a result, we are automating our success.

In the pages ahead, I will lay out a set of actions for eating Keto in the form of a simple system. Plug and play, rinse and repeat, heat and eat with your air fryer! By front-loading your limited willpower with a simple plan, you will avoid making off-plan buying decisions as your week gets busier and more stressful. You will find you save money and time. Better yet, you will avoid having to make any decisions relating to food and drink for the week ahead. This set routine ultimately leads to a more successful and satisfying life.

Why do so many "successful eaters" eat the same foods every day?

We now know that what we eat and drink takes thousands of decisions per week… unless we have a system to reduce them. I borrowed from the capsule wardrobe concept to create my 7

Day Meal Capsule System in the form of this simple Challenge to help reduce your daily food decisions and to automate your willpower. Can I mess up a perfectly good week of eating without a plan? Yes, of course, I can. Even though I have been eating this way for years, I have repeatedly proven that I can screw this up, even while writing this book on how *not to screw this up*. Your system is only guaranteed to work if you use it. We all need systems in our lives.

For the past few weeks, as I attempt to edit the sentences that will become this book, I have struggled with my own food choices. Why? The list goes on and on… I got busy… it's the holiday season… I was too focused on writing... The hamster wheel in my brain was anxiously spinning and spinning out of control on some days. You know how it goes with life's many distractions and stressors, right? I'm preaching to the choir again.

Real life with plenty of stress happens to all of us—*that's life*. During the holidays, my lifestyle became a roller coaster of eating keto one day and then high-carb meals the next day. Side Note: I strongly dislike roller coasters. I'd consume pizza and cookies (hundreds of processed carbs) one day and then eat steak and eggs (almost no carbs) the next day. At times, I was even mainlining large amounts of sugar-filled things, like my daughter's delicious Christmas treats that she made to give to her friends as gifts. Why? Because they were there and looked and smelled amazing, I had no plan for the week, and I ran out of willpower. I didn't bother to put anything in my calendar about how I intended to fuel my body. I would forget what day it was and even lose track of time some days. I did not have a plan in place for buying the right foods or making the meals... I just kind of winged it. The beginning of the end, as they say. *Fail to plan, plan to fail, they also say.*

Enter random eating out of convenience, and add in some emotional eating, too. To compound the bad food decisions, I made sure to sprinkle in drinking a bit too much alcohol, too. It's easy to default to someone else's plan for you if you don't have one. It's also just as easy to follow your plan if you have one. Not choose your hard. Choose your easy!

Why not just wing it?

You have heard of the pre-flight checklist for airline pilots, right? This required checklist is another proven system. A pilot relies on a proven system, a checklist of actions to fly a plane safely every single time. A surgeon depends on a proven system of actions to perform successful surgeries every single time. These highly skilled professionals don't leave anything to chance (thank God) when flying a plane or performing any delicate surgeries. Can you imagine a surgeon just "winging it" on some delicate brain surgery?! We must implement the same strategy in our lives regarding how we want to fuel our bodies for the same results.

Q: *How long does it take to form a habit?*
A: *It varies widely!*

According to a 2009 study published in the *European Journal of Social Psychology,* a person takes 18 to 254 days to form a new habit. The study also concluded that, on average, it takes 66 days for a new behavior to become automatic. The 2009 study highlighted a range of variables in habit forming that make it impossible to establish a "one size fits all" answer. For example, certain habits take longer to create. As demonstrated in the study, many participants found it easier to adopt the habit of drinking a glass of water at breakfast than to do 50 sit-ups after their morning coffee.

The science is inconclusive on how long it takes to form a habit. As the study above proved, it varies according to the habit in question and by each individual. Again, there are no one-size-fits-all answers here. It makes sense, as we are all unique individuals with many glorious differences. We are humans, after all, not robots. We all have different goals, personalities, bodies, and tastes. We are deciding and committing to specific actions by putting them in our calendar to ensure we do them. We always fall back on the systems we put in place.

Why just 7 days in this Challenge?

A system, by design, will kick in for everyone on day one—there is no need to wait any days at all to have this work. A habit system entered into your non-negotiable calendar ensures that your behaviors, and then your results, become automatic. Habits repeated in the form of a system create momentum.

"I think of momentum as the fertilizer for growing lasting habits."

Looking and feeling noticeably better will create momentum for you quickly. This quick momentum you will feel in just seven days will inspire you to continue week in and week out with this eating outline if you see it's working for you. Our brains crave structure, familiarity, and order... systems give them just that.

"Change your habits, change your life, change the world!"

Having habit-based systems in our lives frees up our mental energy to make better quality-of-life decisions and provides more mental capacity to make positive things happen for us and those we support! What will you get done with all this extra time and mental capacity freed up by having systems in place!? *The sky's the limit!*

Eating with a purpose, *your purpose*

You don't need to be a great cook to put these simple ingredient meals together. All the recipes in the Challenge are simple, healthy, low-carb, and delicious. By design, they share healthy fat and protein ingredients to keep you feeling full. The simple recipes have "done for you" calculated carb counts under the daily limit (25 Grams net carbs) to get you into ketosis and burning fat instead of sugar as soon as possible. Net carbs are the total carbs minus any Grams of fiber in the food. *It's all done for you here!*

I provide the answers to the question that comes up every day, again and again, 1,589 times 7 days a week...

"What am I going to eat today!?"

5

WEEKLY MEAL PREP IS TOO COMPLEX

Is Keto just too hard?

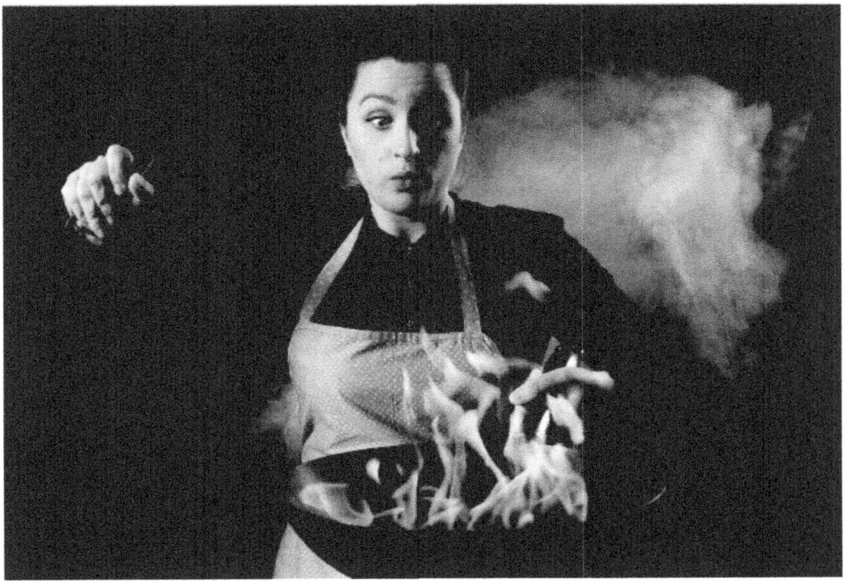

What if I'm not good at cooking or I just really hate to cook?
What if I'm on a limited budget?
What if I'm just too busy?

The Keto Diet, or any diet, can be too hard. Complex definitions, confusing opinions from "trusted sources," fancy, elaborate, sixteen or more ingredient recipes, and of course, the complicated tracking apps and spreadsheets to help us count and track all these crazy things. It's all a bit much, right? It's totally understandable why most people may believe that dieting, including Keto, is just way too hard! With all of this, it's understandable why a large percentage of people just quit in disgust.

I hear all of these concerns and many more... I've addressed each one of these valid concerns with this simple, affordable, 7 Day Air Fryer Challenge. I've honed this simple keto meal plan for the week down to the Minimum Effective Keto Diet. It's the simplest version I've ever seen. Simple, yet highly effective for anyone that has found Keto to be too hard to do in the past.

Are Keto recipes too complex?

Many that you see online on social media posts sure are! This is yet another big reason why people may think the Keto Diet is just too hard, and they are not wrong. Just search Instagram if you want to see the most incredible, gourmet dishes that come with an impossible-to-find list of ingredients, and that are even harder to make. Discouraging? You bet it is!

Fancy, complex, Instagram Keto food pics:

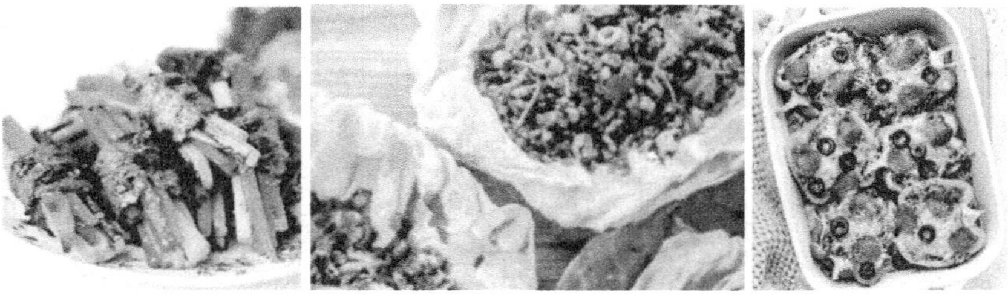

Many of these recipes have sixteen or more ingredients and include ingredients that you can't even pronounce... Some recipes require hours of prep and cooking time if you hope to prepare these fancy Keto dishes in your kitchen. *Is this realistically sustainable on a busy school or work night?* Not if you want to try to get to sleep before midnight... I prefer to be in my bed at 9:30, thank you!

"Ain't nobody got time for that!"

This is why people and many so-called "trusted sources" bash the Keto Diet (or at least don't get on board with it) for it being too restrictive, complex, and just too hard to sustain... and they would be right. But it's just short-sighted to throw away the potential lifestyle success that the keto diet offers so many of us. It just needs to be made easy! We make it easy here, so you can actually do it and then see if it works for you long term.

Here is a pic from my social media feed of a simple-to-make, delicious ribeye steak cooked in the air fryer. Nothing complex to see here... a steak, some seasoning, topped with butter at the end. *Simple Perfection!*

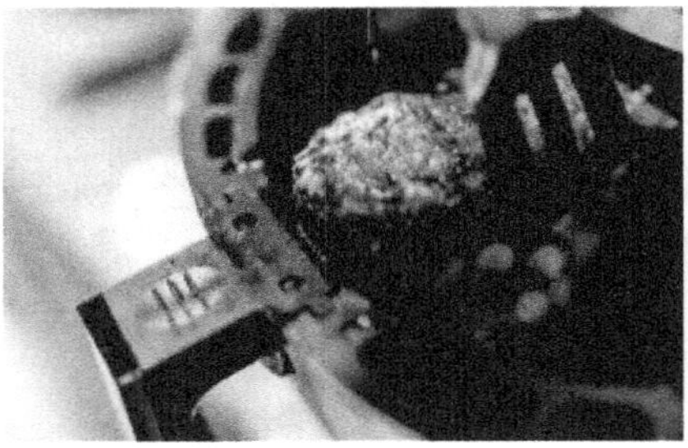

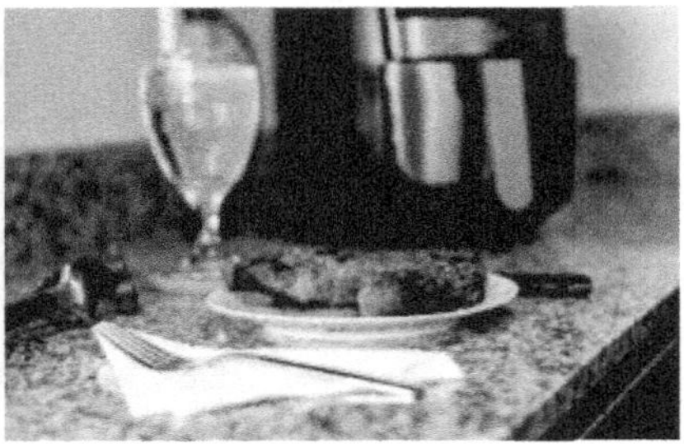

Challenge FB group page, please join the Challenge Community via the link or QR code below!

https://www.facebook.com/ketolifeupgrade

Is Keto too expensive?

Keto does not need to be expensive. In fact, you can buy quality sourced foods at value prices in any market if you know what to look for. I will teach you what to look for and how not to spend too much! Join our Challenge Facebook Group for real-time updates when I am out shopping in the market, and I find great deals on quality keto foods. I share these great deals, frequently found in the national food chains that are in most of our client's markets.

From now on, your grocery store trips should never be random or impulsive. You will always have a plan for your weekly shopping and of course, your list of exactly what to buy to make your meals. There are sales on quality food all the time, and it pays to shop the sales. The cost savings all add up! I frequent certain national retailers, like Aldi, that combine quality sourced foods with discounted prices. Another store I just love is Costco! Costco has a great corporate food-buying team that always seems to source great quality foods and negotiates down the prices for their members. They run a monthly savings offer on select items, too, so you can stock up if these align with your Keto food plan. They have a special membership card that gives you cash back on purchases you can use to save even more, with money rebated at the end of every year. An added benefit: You can even return food if you get it home, try it, and don't love it for any reason... No questions asked! As I stated earlier, we vote with our dollars, and when we do, Big Food will continue to add more Keto foods for us to buy. We are affecting this positive change slowly but surely!

I will bet that your weekly food cost for this Challenge will be less than you normally spend on your current (baseline) diet. You may not have been shopping with a plan before, and this extra focus alone will help you shave expenses. You won't be buying things on impulse or making bad decisions without a plan in hand. I bet you will save more than enough in week one of your Challenge to pay for this course!

Another benefit of eating Keto... you are not feeling like you are starving all the time; therefore, you don't need to eat as many meals or as much food. You will feel more satisfied eating quality fats and proteins, and you can go longer between meals as a result. Eating indeed becomes "optional." Soon you will be able to skip meals when you feel like it once you switch over to burning fat for your fuel source. Less waste, more nutrients in your foods, with fewer meals needed. These changes will result in you spending less money over time with Keto. *More wins for you!*

Not enough time (or any desire) to cook

Listen, friends, I'm a foodie... I love to experiment in the kitchen with different recipes. I love to create and sample all kinds of new meals when I have the time. But like many of you, I don't always have the time or feel like cooking, either. Over the years of eating Keto, I have tested many low-carb recipes and cooking methods. You name it, and I've tried it. From grilling to baking in the oven, to the Instant Pot, Crock Pot, and stove pot on the stove... The list goes on and on... most of us are just too darn busy these days to spend lots of time and effort on cooking. If and when cooking food becomes inconvenient, then it becomes not sustainable.

The Air Fryer Revolution!

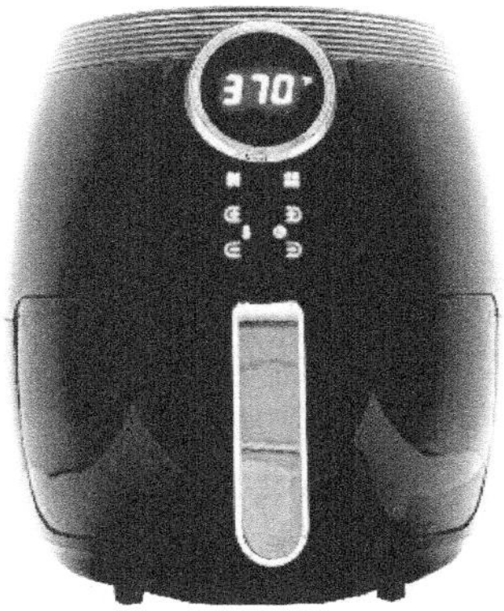

A small convection oven for any small counter space. It's hard to mess up cooking with an air fryer, and it takes minimal time and effort. It's perfect for the theme in this course, *simple Keto... less really can be more.*

Plug in the air fryer, and plug into this system!

"Plug in the air fryer, and plug into this system!" This could have been the title of this book. I must admit, I'm obsessed with my air fryer, and I'm really okay with that. That's how much I love my air fryer for preparing great-tasting, low-carb foods! I didn't make that the title, but I have made the air fryer the only appliance you need to make all the simple recipes in this Challenge.

In this 7 Day Air Fryer Challenge, I provide you with the simple directions to season, heat, and eat everything with this one very affordable, easy-to-use kitchen appliance. Anyone can use it anywhere you have an electric outlet and two square feet of space.

Why the air fryer? Kind of like the Keto Diet over the decades; what's old is new again. It's a convection oven that cooks by circulating dry heat but is much smaller and very portable. I've experimented with many cooking methods over the years. I like to test new things, and I usually get excited about a new appliance when I first get it, and then... it ends up collecting dust in the basement, never to be used again. *Not true with the air fryer!* As I started to take notes for this book over a year ago, I was well into my obsession with this incredibly effective appliance. It really is the *minimum effective applianc*e for cooking great-tasting food in less time and with easy cleanup, too. It’s almost foolproof for getting great-tasting results.

The growing list of why I love my air fryer:

☑ It's simple to cook with, basically a temp and a time. It's tough to mess anything up.

☑ “Set it and forget it!” You can multitask while cooking your food or just sit back and relax.

☑ It cooks with dry heat, making you less likely to lose key nutrients from your food.

☑ Reheating leftovers is just as easy, and they taste just as good, if not better!

☑ Crispy vegetables taste great! *Who knew?!*

☑ Burgers (or any meat) finish crisp on the outside while remaining tender on the inside.

☑ Amazing bacon cooking method with less splatter mess.

☑ Less energy is used less heat in the house, and less cost.
☑ Time saver! Foods cook very fast.
☑ Easy to clean up.
☑ Ideal for small spaces like a camper, a condo, or apartment living.
☑ Replaces many other appliances, which gives you back even more space in your pantry or kitchen.
☑ It uses little to no oil. I add healthy oils on top of most foods to help them brown, plus extra nutrients/flavor are in the healthy fats like extra virgin olive oil.

Air fryer tips

✔ Don't spray the air fryer basket with any oils before adding food.
✔ Buy a larger air fryer if you have the space and cook for more than 2 people. Still, minimal spaced needed.
✔ Remember to flip your food over or shake the basket at the 50 percent cook time mark. This doesn't have to be exact timing, either.
✔ Don't crowd the air fryer basket by putting too much food in at once. Less crowding allows the heat to circulate around food for more even cooking and faster cooking times, too.
✔ Thaw out your meat for at least twenty-four hours in the fridge in a sealed bag or container before cooking. This will save you time when cooking, it will help cook your food more evenly, and everything will taste better.
✔ You don't have to thaw frozen veggies before cooking.

They cook from frozen just fine, but thawed is a much faster cook time. I usually buy frozen vegetables as the micronutrients are locked in more than the "fresh" produce. If you are in season and have access to a Farmer's Market for your produce, great! If not, you risk getting far less than fresh produce, as it has to travel a long way to get to your grocery store.

This is a Challenge about investing... *Investing in YOU with your food choices!*

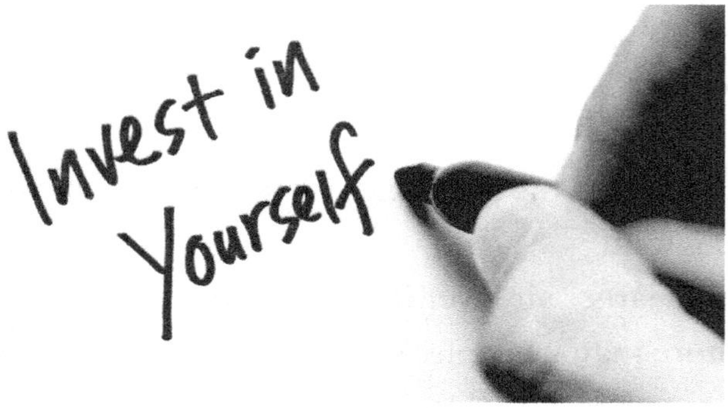

What could be more important than investing in your future health and happiness?! You will be systematically investing in your health and vitality every week. Your stock picks? Your food and drinks. My clients see me as their food market advisor for easy keto success at the lowest cost. Week after week, you will be compounding your future positive health returns. No more food market manipulation for you! We can and will make the food marketplace work for us!! You are, in effect, planning for your future health and wellness by what goes into your grocery cart, into your fridge, and into your body.

Some of the stocked markets you will be investing in for your health!

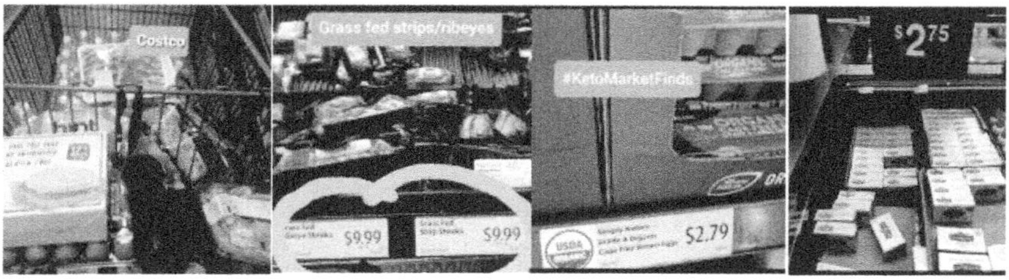

I advise you to invest in different types of "stocked markets" for huge returns on your health and happiness. I look for healthy, quality-sourced, low-carb foods, and it's even better when we are down with a discount! It does not have to be expensive to live a healthy Keto lifestyle! It won't be with this Challenge. Even if you are in your 80s, you can invest in looking and feeling better starting today! It's never too late to start investing in YOU! *You deserve it!*

It's not normal to be fat and sick at any age! Many have been conditioned to believe this is an inevitable part of the biological aging process. I could not disagree more, and I flat-out refuse to believe it's "normal" to be fat and sick at any age. Becoming obese and staying that way is super expensive over time! Being obese is a very bad return on your investment financially and, worse, on your quality of life. We are talking about poor quality of life and super high disease care costs. I'm thrilled you have decided to take action and take control of this positive outcome for yourself!

6

YOUR SIMPLE 7 DAY RECIPES

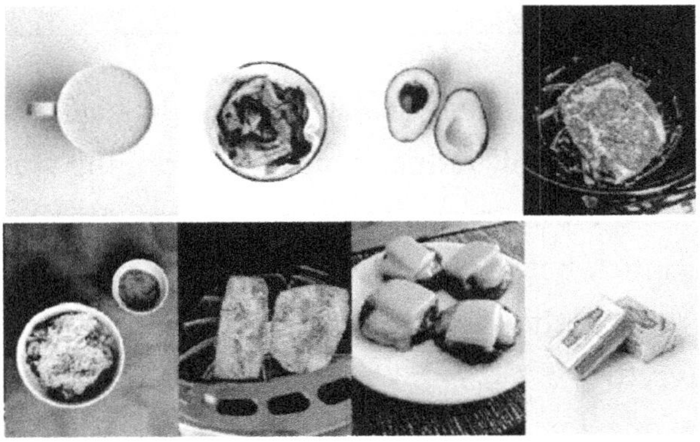

Here I will give you the simple to make, air fryer "recipes" for your Challenge week ahead. Really, it's the simple steps to *heat 'n' eat* your meals. It's hardly cooking, but the results are just as good, if not better. We make the Keto lifestyle easy right here. One of my favorite quotes and foods:

"When in doubt, eat more steak!"

Use any digital or print calendar that works for you. Google has a free calendar that is easy to use with your free Gmail account sign-up if you still need to get a free Gmail account.

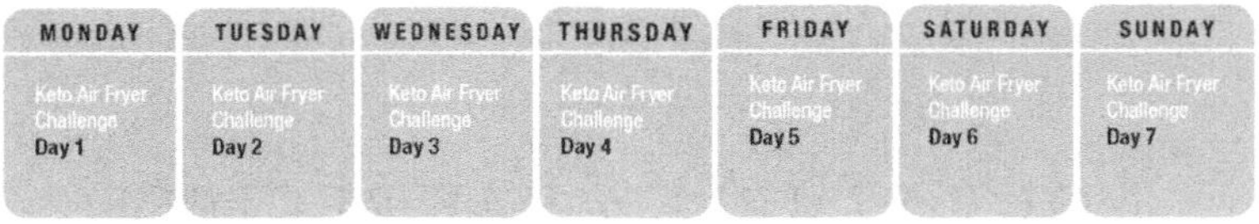
MONDAY
Keto Air Fryer Challenge Day 1
TUESDAY
Keto Air Fryer Challenge Day 2
WEDNESDAY
Keto Air Fryer Challenge Day 3
THURSDAY
Keto Air Fryer Challenge Day 4
FRIDAY
Keto Air Fryer Challenge Day 5
SATURDAY
Keto Air Fryer Challenge Day 6
SUNDAY
Keto Air Fryer Challenge Day 7

I recommend taking your next day's Challenge foods out of your freezer and thawing them in the fridge for 24 hours as a regular habit.

Put foods in a gallon-sized sealable plastic bag as needed in the fridge. Doing this will reduce your food cooking time, and it's easier to season non-frozen food, as the seasoning will stick to your food much better. An added benefit to thawing foods out ahead of time is that you ensure even cooking results. It just tastes better, too!

Start each Challenge Day off with some hydration with added electrolytes.

Starting your day with hydration and electrolytes can have a range of benefits for your health and well-being, including all of the following.

Hydration

Drinking water in the morning can help to rehydrate your body after a night of sleep when you may not have consumed any fluids for several hours. This habit can help to boost your energy levels, improve your mental clarity, and support your overall health and well-being.

Electrolyte balance

Electrolytes are essential minerals that help to regulate many of the body's functions, including fluid balance, nerve function, and muscle contractions. Starting your day with a source of electrolytes, such as a sports drink or electrolyte powder, can help to replenish any electrolytes lost during the night and support optimal health and performance.

Digestion

Drinking morning water can help stimulate your digestive system and support healthy bowel movements. This habit can help to reduce bloating, constipation, and other digestive issues and support overall gut health.

Metabolism

Staying hydrated and maintaining electrolyte balance can also support a healthy metabolism, as many metabolic processes rely on adequate hydration and electrolyte levels. This habit can help to support healthy weight management and overall health.

Skin health

Drinking water and electrolytes can also support healthy skin, as hydration is essential for maintaining skin elasticity and preventing dryness and wrinkles.

In addition to these benefits, research has also shown that dehydration and electrolyte imbalances can have a range of adverse effects on the body, including headaches, fatigue, muscle weakness, and cognitive impairment. By starting your day with hydration and electrolytes, you can help to prevent these negative effects and support your overall health and well-being.

Fill up a large drinking glass with filtered water, add a teaspoon of Redmond's Sea Salt, squeeze in a quarter of a lemon, and drink it down. That will give your body some needed electrolytes and wake up your system for the day! Next, I highly recommend enjoying your Keto coffee or tea. This coffee tastes divine, and this healthy habit will spike your ketones first thing every morning! Drinking this will also curb your appetite so you can go longer before consuming your first meal of the day. The mix of organic coffee and these quality fat ingredients will also boost your cognitive functioning and should increase your energy levels as you start your day. You will see this simple recipe for Keto coffee below. You can get Redmond's Sea Salt, Bulletproof MCT Oil, and other recommended Challenge products on the resources page on my website for easy ordering and delivery right to your house.

These Challenge simple recipes, indeed, are the Minimum Effective Keto Diet!

Here is the 7 Day snapshot of each day's meals, followed by the simple recipes to make each one.

Monday (Challenge Day 1) Foods: 8 Grams of carbs (1 cup of Broccoli)

Keto Coffee, Boiled Eggs, Bacon, Steak, Broccoli (eat as much as you want of everything except limit Broccoli to 1 Cup).

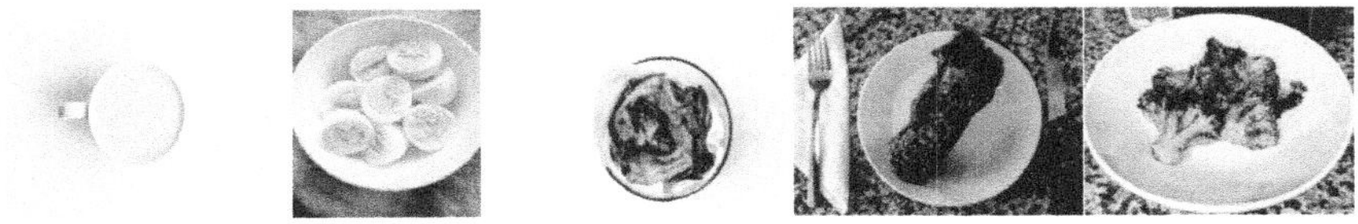

Tuesday (Challenge Day 2) Foods: 8 Grams of carbs (1 cup Brussels)

Keto Coffee, Boiled Eggs, Sausage, Salmon, Brussels Sprouts (eat as much as you want of everything except limit Brussels Sprouts to 1 Cup).

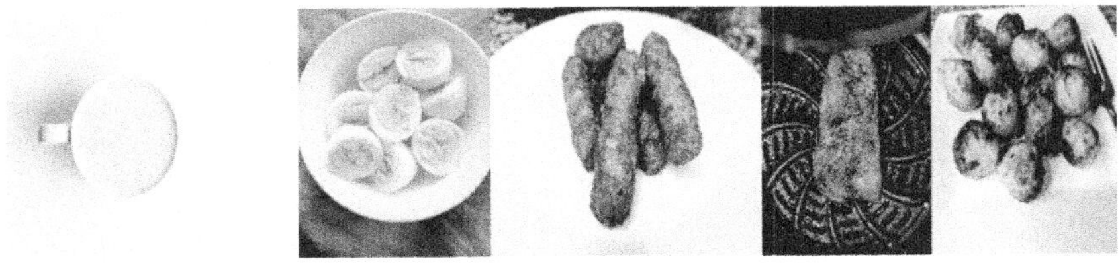

Wednesday (Challenge Day 3) Foods: 8 Grams of carbs (1 large Avocado)

Keto Coffee, Boiled Eggs, Cheese, Cheeseburgers, Avocado (eat as much as you want of everything except limit to 1 large Avocado).

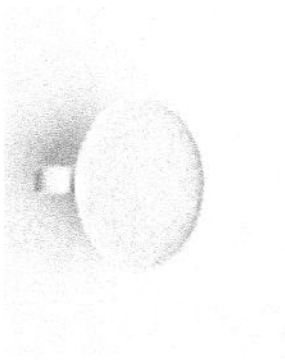 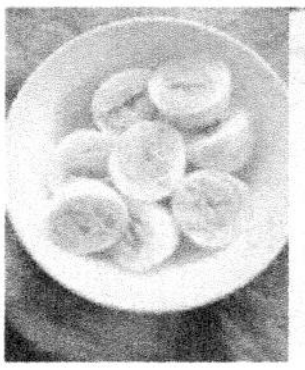 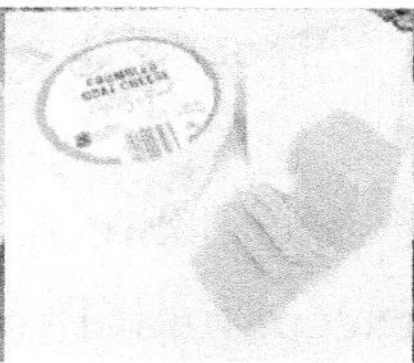 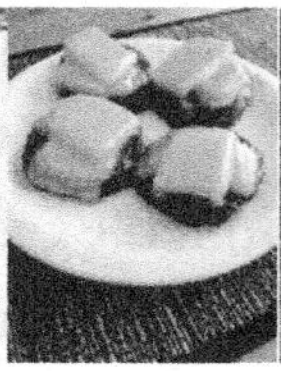 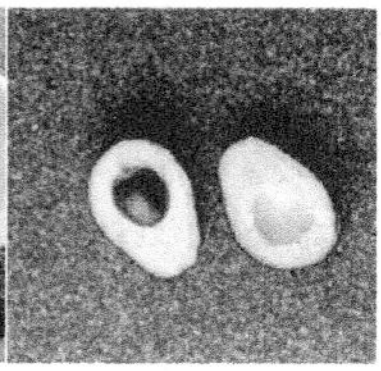

Thursday (Challenge Day 4) Foods: 8 Grams of carbs (1 cup of Olives)

Keto Coffee, Boiled Eggs, Bacon, Lamb, Olives (eat as much as you want of everything except limit Olives to 1 Cup).

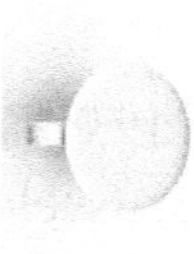 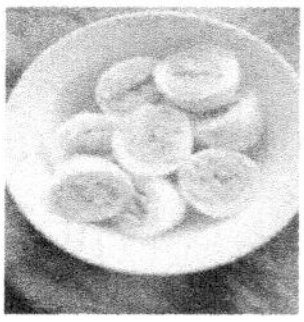 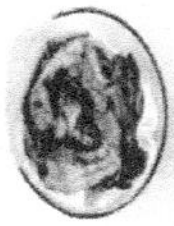 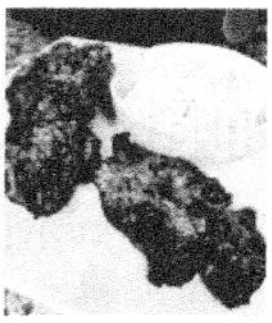 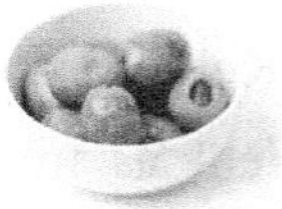

Friday (Challenge Day 5) Foods: 10 Grams of carbs (1 cup Sauerkraut)

Keto Coffee, Boiled Eggs, Sausage, Brats and Sauerkraut (eat as much as you want of everything except limit Sauerkraut to 1 Cup).

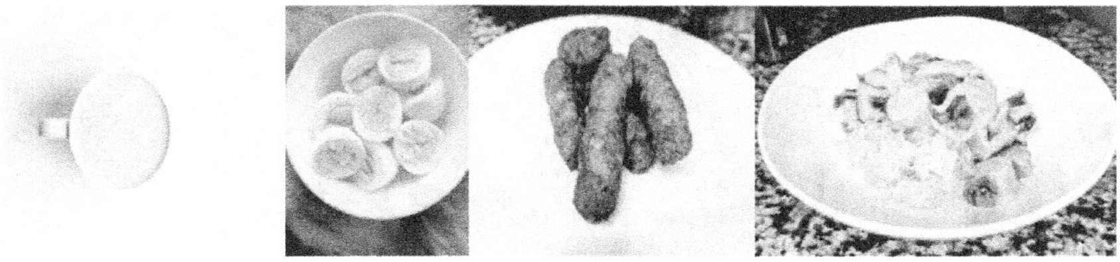

Saturday (Challenge Day 6) Foods: 6 Grams of carbs (1 cup Broccoli)

Keto Coffee, Boiled Eggs, Cheese, Chicken, Broccoli (eat as much as you want of everything except limit Broccoli to 1 Cup).

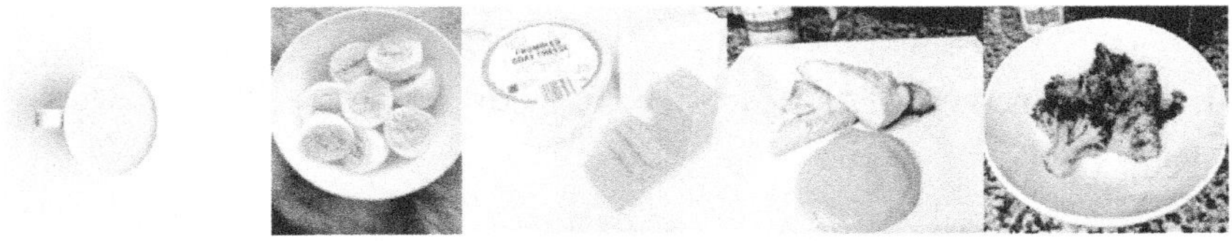

Sunday (Challenge Day 7) Foods: 8 Grams of carbs (1 cup Brussels sprouts)

Keto Coffee, Steak, Boiled Eggs, Salmon, Brussels Sprouts (eat as much as you want of everything except limit brussels sprouts to 1 cup).

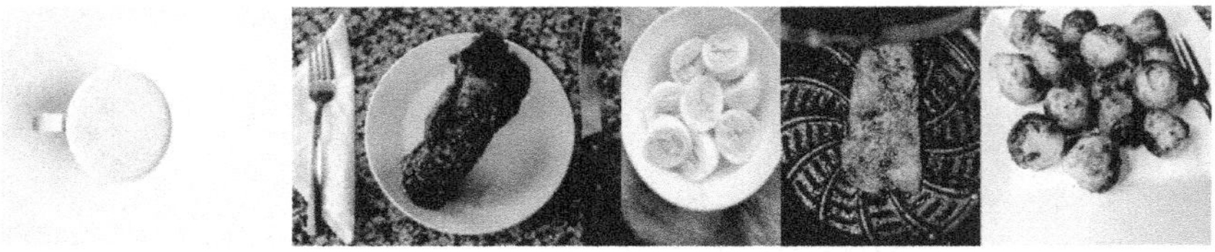

Keto Coffee/Keto Tea
Carbs: 0 Grams
Time to make: 5 minutes

Ingredients

1 cup of brewed organic coffee or 1 cup of steeped black or green tea
1 tablespoon unsalted Kerrygold butter
1 tablespoon Brain Octane MCT Oil

Simple Directions

1. Add your butter and MCT oil to the blender cup.
2. Pour a cup of brewed coffee or tea into your Nuribullet blender cup.

3. Blend for 20 seconds.
4. Pour back into the coffee cup and enjoy! If you like your coffee hotter, heat it in the microwave after blending it for 15 seconds.

TIP

I recommend enjoying one to two cups daily, 90 minutes after waking to start your day off strong. You can add a cup of coffee or tea later in the day to help curb your appetite. If it's after 2:00 p.m., I suggest choosing a decaffeinated version so it doesn't disturb your sleep later that night.

Air Fryer Boiled Eggs (no water needed)
Carbs: 0 Grams
Time to cook: 17 minutes

Ingredients

Up to 8 eggs at a time
Redmond's Kosher Sea Salt to taste
Ground pepper to taste

Simple Directions

1. Place up to 8 eggs in your air fryer basket.
2. Cook on 250°F temperature setting; set the timer for 17 minutes for hard-boiled.
3. Place cooked eggs into an ice-water-filled bowl for 3 minutes to make the shells come off easily when peeling.
4. Peel, season, and eat.

TIP

You can store extra eggs in your glass Pyrex containers for snacking on at any time or for the next day's meals.

Bacon
Carbs: 0 Grams
Time to cook: 6 minutes

Ingredients

6–8 strips of pre-cooked bacon

Simple Directions

1. Place 6–8 strips of bacon at a time in the air fryer basket at 400°F temperature setting.
2. Set cook timer for 6 minutes, flipping with tongs halfway through. Cook a little longer if you prefer your bacon crispier.

TIP

It's a little more money to buy the pre-cooked bacon, but it's well worth it! Less mess to clean up, as much of the grease was cooked off already, and a much faster cook time, too.

Pork Sausage Links
Carbs: 2 Grams per 6 sausage links
Time to cook: 8 minutes

Ingredients

6–8 pre-cooked frozen sausage links

Simple Directions

1. Place 6–8 pre-cooked frozen sausage links in the air fryer basket at 400°F temperature setting.
2. Set the cook timer for 8 minutes and start. Shake the air fryer basket a couple of times at the 4-minute mark to ensure even cooking.

TIP

It's also a little more money to buy pre-cooked sausage, but again, it's worth it! Less mess to clean up as much of the grease was cooked off already, and faster time to heat and enjoy your sausage links!

Ribeye Steak
Carbs: 0 Grams
Time to cook: 14 minutes

Ingredients

1 ribeye or New York Strip steak
1 tablespoon salted Kerrygold butter
1 tablespoon extra virgin olive oil
1 teaspoon Montreal Steak Seasoning (optional)
1 teaspoon Redmond's Kosher Sea Salt

Ground pepper to taste

Simple Directions

1. Drizzle olive oil on the steak, add seasonings, and then rub seasonings into the steak.
2. Repeat on the other side of the steak.
3. Set your timer for 7 minutes and temperature setting to 400°F. Flip your steak with tongs at 7 minutes of cooking time to ensure even cooking. For medium rare, cook 7 minutes per side per inch-thick cut of meat.
4. Allow your steak to "rest" (set on a cutting board with tin foil over it) for 5 minutes after cooking is complete. This resting period allows the steak's juices to redistribute into the meat, so it tastes incredible!
5. While your steak is resting, add butter on top of your steak to melt it down.

TIP

You don't want to overcook your steak, whatever that means to you. I recommend setting the AF cook timer for 7 minutes per side, per inch thickness of your steak. Check the steak once the timer goes off to see if it is done enough for you. You can always add minutes if you want it more done. Of course, you can't un-cook the food if you go too long.

Cheeseburgers

Carbs: 0 Grams

Time to cook: 10 minutes

Ingredients

2 burger patties at a time
2 thick slices of cheddar cheese
1 teaspoon Redmond's Sea Salt
Ground pepper to taste

Simple Directions

1. Add frozen patties to the air fryer basket, set to 400°F temperature setting.
2. Cook for 10 minutes, flipping with tongs at the 5-minute mark.
3. Add seasonings after you flip burgers, as it will stick better to the burger.

TIP

Once the timer goes off, top your burgers with cheese and allow them to melt in the AF basket for up to a minute.

Salmon
Carbs: 0 Grams
Time to cook: 15 minutes

Ingredients

2 boneless, skinless salmon filets (thaw frozen salmon in fridge 24 hours before cooking)
4 lemon slices
2 tablespoons extra virgin olive oil
1 teaspoon paprika
1 teaspoon Redmond's Kosher Sea Salt
Ground pepper to taste

Simple Directions

1. Slice a lemon into 4 slices and place the cut slices in the AF basket, as seen in the image below.
2. Lay the salmon filets on top of the lemon slices (this infuses flavor and better heat circulation for your salmon to cook).
3. Drizzle extra virgin olive oil on filets, and add all the seasonings to the top side of your salmon.
4. Set the timer for 15 minutes, and heat at 400°F temperature setting (no need to flip).

TIP

Plan to thaw your frozen salmon filets in the fridge overnight. By thawing them out 1 day before cooking, the salmon filets are easier to season, will cook more evenly, and will need less cooking time for you to enjoy.

Brussels Sprouts
Carbs: 1 cup: 8 Grams (per 1 cup of Brussels sprouts)
Time to cook: 12–14 minutes

Ingredients

1 bag of frozen Brussels sprouts
1 tablespoon extra virgin olive oil
1 teaspoon Redmond's Kosher Sea Salt
Ground pepper to taste

Simple Directions

1. Cut open the Brussels sprouts bag, and add extra virgin olive oil and salt and pepper to the sprouts in the bag.
2. Close the top of the bag and shake it a few times to coat it with your oil and seasonings.
3. Place Brussels sprouts into the air fryer basket, set to 375°F temperature.

4. Cook the Brussels sprouts for 12–14 minutes till they are done to your liking (longer time for crispy texture). Shake the air fryer basket a couple of times during the cooking time to ensure even cooking.

TIP

Thaw overnight in the fridge to reduce air fryer cooking time.

Broccoli
Carbs: 1 cup: 8 Grams (per 1 cup broccoli)
Time to cook: 12–14 minutes

Ingredients

1 bag of broccoli
1 tablespoon extra virgin olive oil
1 teaspoon Redmond's Sea Salt
Ground pepper to taste

Simple Directions

1. Cut open a bag of broccoli, and add extra virgin olive oil and salt and pepper to the broccoli in the bag.

2. Close the top of the bag and shake it a few times to coat it with your oil and seasonings.
3. Place the broccoli into the air fryer basket, set to 375°F temperature.
4. Cook the broccoli 12–14 minutes till they are done to your liking (longer for crispier broccoli), shaking the basket a couple of times during the cooking time to ensure even cooking.

TIP

Thaw overnight in the fridge to reduce air fryer cooking time.

Brat Bowl with Sauerkraut, Mustard, and Onions (toppings optional)

Carbs: 0 Grams with just bratwurst

Carbs: 9 Grams (with 1 cup sauerkraut and 2 tbsp onions)

Time to cook: 8 minutes

Ingredients

Up to 4 pre-cooked bratwurst sausages at a time

1 cup sauerkraut

2 tablespoons chopped onion (optional)

Mustard (optional)

Simple Directions

1. Add 2–4 pre-cooked brats to the air fryer basket, set to 375°F temperature setting.
2. Cook for 5 minutes; give the air fryer basket a shake 3 minutes in to help them heat through evenly.
3. Chop up finished brats and add to a large bowl. Top with sauerkraut, chopped onions, and mustard.

Leg of Lamb Steaks
Carbs for lamb: 0 Grams
Carbs: 1 Gram (per 1 Tbsp Tzatziki Sauce)
Time to cook: 16 minutes

Ingredients

2 legs of lamb "steaks" cut to 1 inch thick
2 tablespoons extra virgin olive oil
2 teaspoons rosemary seasoning
2 teaspoons minced garlic
1 teaspoon Redmond's Sea Salt
Ground pepper to taste
2 tablespoons Tzatziki Sauce

Simple Directions

1. Cut 1-inch thick "steak" slices off the leg of lamb. Seal and store the rest in the fridge for later use. You will have plenty extra for more meals.
2. Drizzle olive oil on both sides of your lamb steak and add garlic and seasonings; rub seasonings into the lamb steak.
3. Cook on 400°F temperature setting. Set the timer for 8 minutes per side per inch thick steak for medium rare, flipping steak with tongs.
4. Let your lamb steaks "rest" for 5 minutes after cooking. Add the Tzatziki Sauce on the side, and enjoy.

Chicken Breast
Carbs: 0 Grams for chicken (low-carb sauces will add a few carbs to your meal)
Time to cook: 18 minutes

Ingredients

2 chicken breasts
Low-carb dipping sauce of choice (read labels for carb count)
1 teaspoon Redmond's Sea Salt
Ground pepper to taste

Simple Directions

1. Cook thawed chicken breasts at 400°F temperature setting for 18 minutes. Flip chicken with tongs at the 9-minute mark.
2. After flipping, season the chicken with salt and pepper to your liking.
3. Add your favorite low-carb sauce to the side for dipping, and enjoy.

TIP

For the juiciest, most tender chicken breasts, the secret is a "wet brine." To "wet brine," immerse your chicken breasts in the ingredients below and place them in the refrigerator for 15 minutes to 2 hours before cooking in your air fryer. This simple process will increase the moisture in the meat and infuse it with flavors, too.

Wet Brine Ingredients: 4 cups water, ¼ cup kosher salt. You can add fresh herbs, minced garlic, or lemon peel for different flavors as you like.

Low-Carb "Keto Condiments"

You can find these condiments in most stores, and many have 2–3 Grams of carbs per serving size, and some will have a little more. Your Challenge daily meals are all set under 10 carbs per day, so you have some room to add these without exceeding 25 Grams of carbs per day.

Remember to read the labels for carb counts and pay attention to the carbs per "serving size."

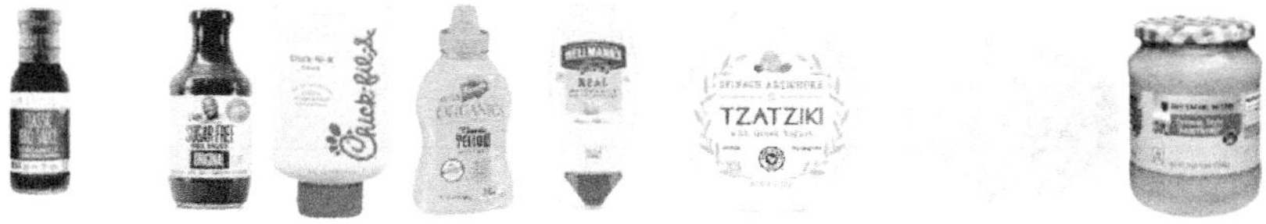

Easy Keto Sides

Kerrygold butter (0 Grams of carbs)
Avocados (8 Grams of carbs per large Avocado)
Olives (8 Grams of carbs per 1 cup)
Cheeses (0 Grams of carbs)

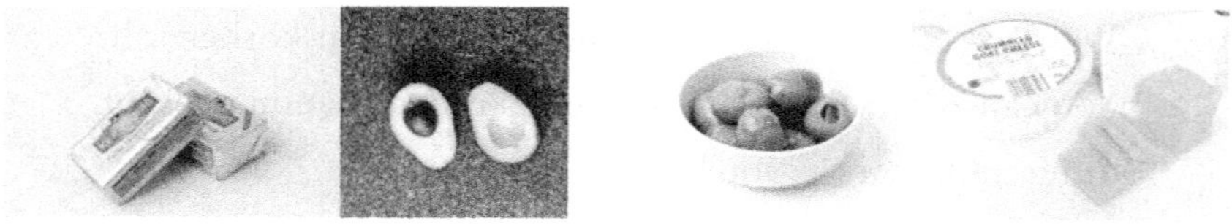

7

CHALLENGE CHECKLIST FOR SUCCESS

Let's get started!!

Here we prepare your mindset and kitchen to ensure you can hit the ground running on your upcoming *7 Day Air Fryer Challenge.*

How to get your Keto Momentum:

➔ Shift from eating the SAD (Standard American Diet) to a healthy Keto Diet. Eating Keto will train your body to burn fat for fuel instead of sugar. *An excellent fuel source upgrade!*

➔ A measurable state of ketosis is achieved when a certain level of ketones is circulating in your blood. *Being in this state will initiate fat loss, reduces food cravings, and produces many other health benefits.*

➔ The carb limit per day is already set for you on this Challenge. *No decisions, no need to track anything.*

This change in how you fuel your body and brain is a HUGE and HEALTHY change! By the end of your first 7 Day Challenge week, you will have your "Keto Momentum" and be on your way to burning fat for fuel instead of sugar! This will get you locked and loaded to automate your success at eating Keto!

Yes, change is hard. Yes, this is different… even a little weird. But the "normal stuff" everyone has been doing is clearly not working. We can see it all around us, and the horrifying data published on the www.cdc.org website further documents that our obesity rates are out of control in this country.

Health condition	Facts
Overweight & Obesity	For more than 25 years, more than half of the adult population has been overweight or obese. Obesity is most prevalent in those ages 40 years and older and in African American adults, and is latest prevalient in adults with higest incomes. 50% Abdominal Obesity In U.S. adults. In 2009-2012. 65% of adult females and 73% of adult males were overweight or obese. In 2009-2012. nearly one in three youth ages 2 to 19 years were overweight or obese.

A declaration is a commitment with teeth! I love this Challenge format because by deciding to do Keto and sharing your intentions, you create accountability in a measurable way. You are plugging into this system to ensure you do this thing! I know you are tired of being fat and sick and feeling like dieting is just too hard! You are making the powerful, life-changing decision here to become a part of this healthy revolution!

How do you ensure that you will take action on your declaration? By putting it in your calendar, and then defending your appointments in the calendar you set because they are your priority. *You and your health are that important!* The calendar appointment is a stronger commitment than a to-do list of any kind. These calendar appointments are your top priorities for the day to make a difference for you and those you love.

"Do. or do not... There is no try."

—Yoda

What are your "whys"?

Most of my clients try Keto for the promise of automatic fat loss and improved body composition. *That's awesome!* I will tell you that many of them, myself included, choose to stay with this lifestyle for those reasons, plus the many other benefits that burning fat for fuel can provide. I experience huge mental health benefits when I eat with a daily carb limit for a week at a time. My brain just works better, as it has more energy in the form of ketones (the brain prefers ketones to glucose for energy). I also notice less anxiety and a better mood, and it helps reduce my ADHD symptoms, too. Being in a state of ketosis also helps my recall, ability to focus on tasks, and my creativity.

Writing down your "whys" for doing something can be a powerful tool for motivation and personal growth. Here are some proven reasons to invest a little time in writing them out:

Clarity

Writing down your "whys" can help you clarify your goals and priorities and articulate them in a way that is meaningful to you. This can make it easier to stay focused and motivated and to make decisions that align with your values and aspirations.

Accountability

When you write down your "whys," you create a tangible reminder of what you're working towards and a commitment to yourself to stay on track. This can help you stay accountable to your goals and take actions consistent with your intentions.

Resilience

Having a clear "why" can help you stay motivated and resilient in the face of challenges and setbacks. By reminding yourself of your deeper purpose and why you're working towards your goals, you can stay focused on the big picture and maintain a sense of perspective and optimism.

Inspiration

Writing down your "whys" can be an inspiring and creative process that can help you connect with your passions, values, and a sense of purpose. By tapping into your inner resources and wisdom, you can find new sources of inspiration and motivation to sustain you over the long term.

Brain function

Writing down your "whys" can have a positive impact on your brain function, memory, and cognition. Research has shown that the act of writing can help to organize your thoughts, clarify your goals, and enhance your ability to learn and remember new information.

Writing down your "whys" for doing something can be a powerful tool for motivation, personal growth, and overall well-being. It can help you clarify your goals, stay accountable, stay resilient, find inspiration, and enhance your brain function.

Invest a few moments to write down what your "whys" are here:

My "whys" are:

____

____

____

____

____

Examples: Fat loss, less bloat, more energy, lower anxiety, disease prevention, anti-aging, reduce inflammation, better focus, look good in a bathing suit, etc.

Kitchen Prep

Clear out your kitchen, including the fridge, freezer, and pantry. The goal here is to get all the non-Keto stuff out of your kitchen and pantry so you won't be tempted to eat it, and most of this stuff is not only high in carbs but in processed seed oils and other junk ingredients that are not at all healthy.

Dump or donate all these foods:

✔ All grain- and sugar-containing foods—bagels, breads, pastas, rice, candy, pastries, cakes, ice cream, chocolates, soda, juices, honey, maple syrup, yogurts, etc.
✔ All starchy vegetables—potatoes, sweet potatoes, parsnips, beans, lentils, chickpeas.
✔ All high-sugar fruits—bananas, pineapples, oranges, apples, grapes, watermelon, mangos.
✔ All sugar/carb-containing beverages.

Your Challenge recommended kitchen items to hit the ground running on Day 1!

Here are all the products you need to kick off your first 7 Day Challenge week, and many more! There is a good chance that you have quite a few of these things on hand already. If you have an Amazon Prime account, most recommended items are delivered for free to your front door. My website resource page, and the Q.R. code to scan with your phone to get right to my resource page, are at the end of this chapter and in the reference section at the end of this book.

Gourmia 7 Quart Air Fryer

I am obsessed with this Gourmia brand air fryer! It's easy to use, and the quality is excellent, too. This one has a larger basket than most air fryers and is dishwasher-safe for easy cleanup.

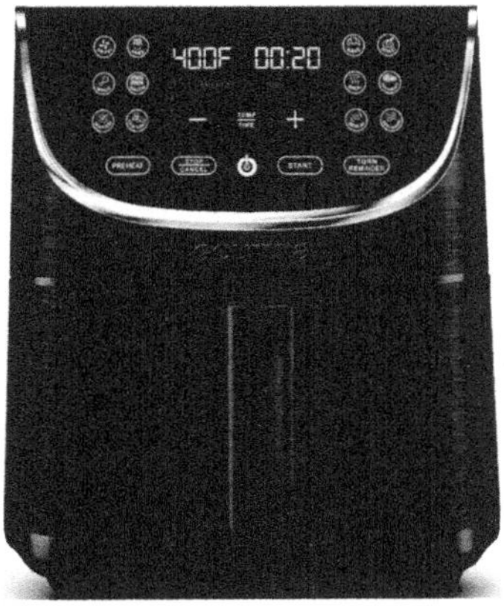

Bulletproof Brain Octane MCT Oil, 32-ounce size

My go-to ingredient to make my morning Keto Coffee. This medium-chain triglyceride oil has a neutral taste, so it mixes well in recipes like dressings or mayo. I always start my day with a cup of this Keto coffee!

We are adding this MCT oil to our coffee, green tea, and any of our foods, even drizzling on top of foods. This healthy oil is an incredible tool for pushing your body into ketosis. It's 14 grams of healthy fat per tablespoon. It's tasteless, too, so it will not impact the flavor of any food or drink. You can add one table-spoon to any drink, including your water. You can even swallow a spoonful straight out of the bottle if you get food cravings, as this oil—which is distilled from the coconut—will curb your cravings and make you feel full, too.

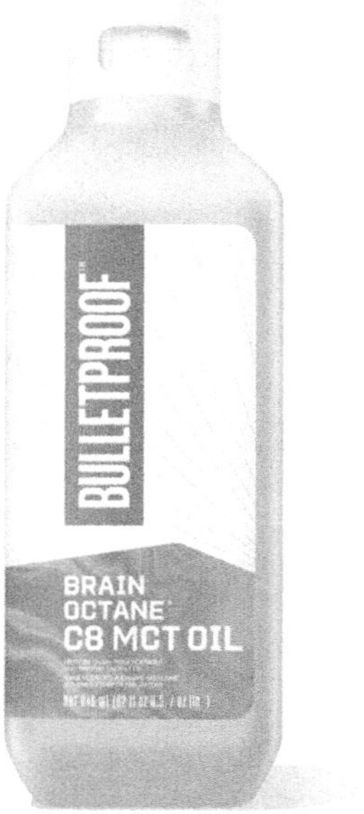

Nutribullet Personal Blender

Best bang for your buck blender that is good quality for the money! It's the perfect size for everything you need and is super easy to clean up, too!

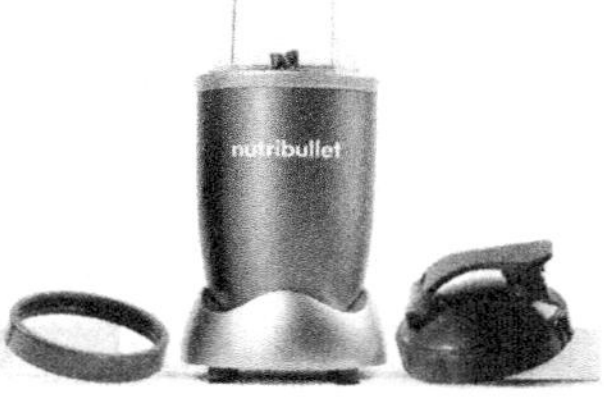

Redmond's Real Sea Salts

Great-tasting seasoning salts for all your Challenge foods. I prefer the "fine" salt with the blue top for recipes and the larger "kosher" salt crystals with the red top for seasoning meats like steak, salmon, and eggs. As an added health bonus, you get extra minerals that your body will appreciate.

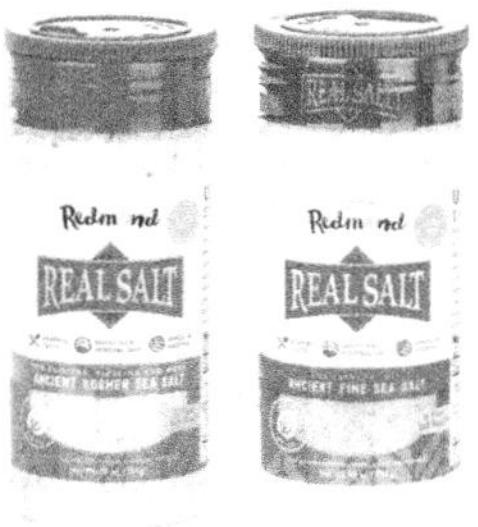

Real Ketone Exogenous Ketone Packets with Electrolytes

When you follow a Ketogenic Diet, your liver makes ketone bodies from fat breakdown from the food you eat. It's like a cheat code for ketosis. There is an additional way to add ready-made ketones by consuming certain supplements. These are called exogenous ketones, as they are made outside of the body. Supplementing your keto diet with exogenous ketones in your water can provide the following benefits:

✔ Consuming these in your water will temporarily raise your blood ketone levels. This means you get more of the beneficial side effects of ketosis! Even when you start your Challenge, and you are still in fat-burning adaptation mode. This can also blunt the effect of consuming too many carbs if you make a mistake—no worries about that on this Challenge. The carb count is set low for you already. Just stick to the blueprint!

✔ Some of you may experience initial flu-like symptoms when transitioning from a high-carb diet to burning fat for fuel. These symptoms are usually temporary but can happen as you are getting off a strong drug known as sugar, so a little detox can be typical. Consuming these can also lessen the Keto Flu's side effects.

✔ Exogenous ketones can suppress the appetite by lowering the hunger hormone ghrelin levels. Consuming these may even suppress your appetite hormones and decrease food cravings, which is always helpful. One recent study showed that appetite decreased between two and four hours after drinking exogenous ketones.

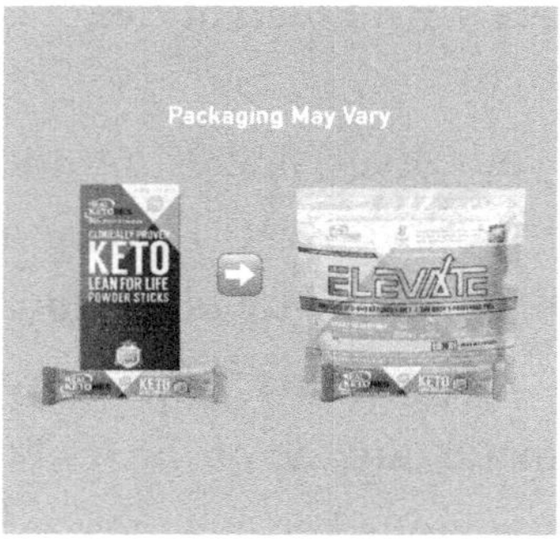

**** Save 10% to 15% more when you set this product up for auto-ship (you'll want a steady supply of this awesome supplement). ****

Silicone Tipped Tongs, 3-Pack

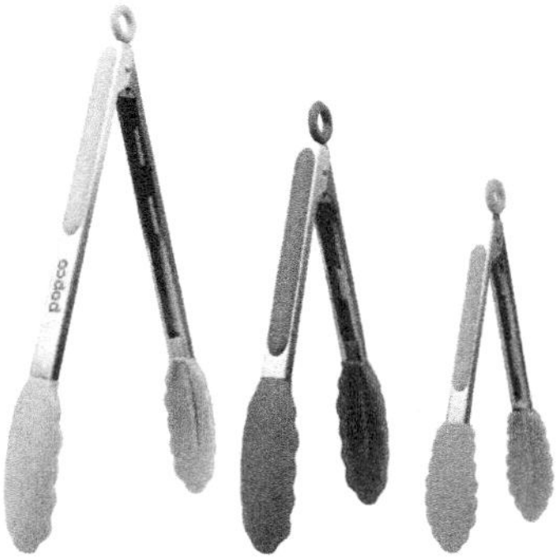

Pyrex Glass Good Storage Container Set, 18 Pieces

This 18-piece set has a great mix of glass food containers to store all your foods in at home and to take with you when you are on the go.

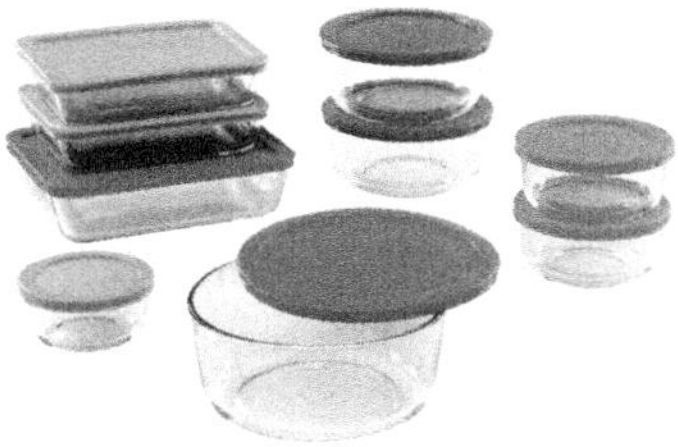

Ziploc Gallon Freezer bags, 2-Pack

Must-have freezer bags for storing food after it's cooked and for thawing meats in the fridge (at least twenty-four hours before heating them up in your air fryer). I recommend thawing most of your Challenge foods for the best outcomes; refer to your *Air Fryer Challenge Recipe* guide for more directions.

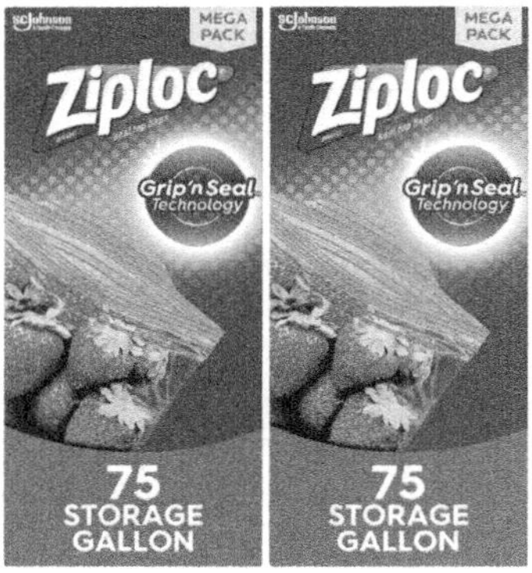

Measuring Spoons - Set of 5

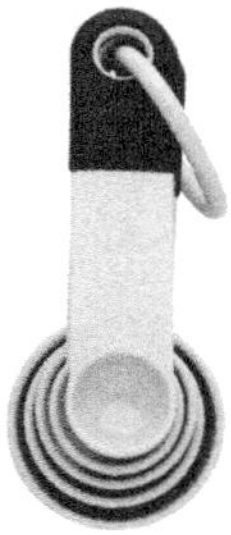

Print off your shopping list here or save it to your phone for easy access. Taking a picture of this page works fine, too. Schedule your grocery shopping trip in your calendar. If you plan for a Monday start, plan to shop Saturday or Sunday, with the list provided here, for your 7 Day Air Fryer Challenge week meals.

Your 7 DAY KETO DIET AIR FRYER Challenge

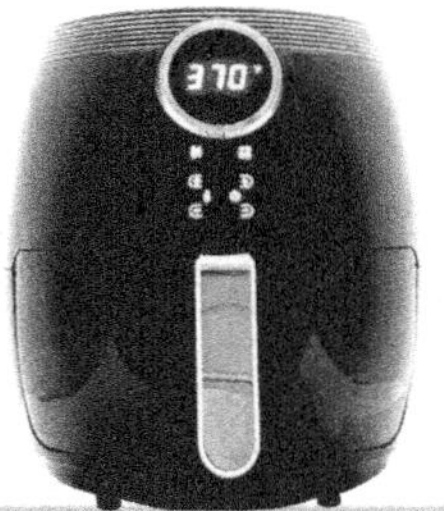

GROCERY LIST

- 1 DOZEN PASTURED EGGS
- 2 LARGE RIBEYE STEAKS
- 1 LEG OF LAMB
- 1 BAG FROZEN CHICKEN BREASTS
- 1 BLOCK KERRYGOLD SALTED BUTTER
- 1 BLOCK KERRYGOLD UNSALTED BUTTER
- 1 PACKAGE OF PRE-COOKED BRATS
- 1 ONION (OPTIONAL)
- 1 BOTTLE OF MUSTARD (OPTIONAL)
- 1 BAG FROZEN SALMON (**COSTCO OR SAM'S CLUB**)
- 1 BOX KEURIG COFFEE CUPS OR COFFEE MAKER GROUND COFFEE (ORGANIC IF POSSIBLE)
- 1 BOX OF GREEN OR BLACK TEA
- 1 32-OUNCE BOTTLE OF BULLETPROOF BRAIN OCTANE OIL (**AMAZON LINK**)
- 1 BAG OF PRE-COOKED BACON
- 1 BAG OF PRE-COOKED BREAKFAST SAUSAGE
- 8 FRESH OR FROZEN HAMBURGER PATTIES
- 1 BLOCK OF CHEDDAR CHEESE
- 1 BAG OF LEMONS
- 1 BOTTLE OF EXTRA VIRGIN OLIVE OIL
- REDMOND SEA SALTS (**AMAZON LINK**)
- 1 CONTAINER OF GROUND PEPPER
- 1 BOTTLE OF PAPRIKA
- 2 BAGS OF FROZEN BROCCOLI
- 2 BAGS OF FROZEN BRUSSELS SPROUTS
- 1 JAR OF SAUERKRAUT
- 1 CONTAINER OF TZATZIKI SAUCE
- 1 JAR OF ROSEMARY SEASONING
- 1 JAR MONTREAL STEAK SEASONING
- 1 SMALL JAR OF MINCED GARLIC
- 1 JAR OF OLIVES
- 1 BAG OF AVOCADOS
- 1 CASE OF PURIFIED WATER (**SMART WATER** FOR LARGER BOTTLES AND GOOD TASTE)
- ANY LOW-CARB DIPPING SAUCES (BBQ, MAYO)

What can I drink on my Challenge?

Keto Coffee (1 to 2 cups daily), green or black teas, sparkling 0-carb flavored waters (Waterloo, Bubly, LeCroix, etc.) If you don't like carbonation, the HINT brand flavored waters are great as they have a fruit flavor with no carbs. Remember to drink plenty of water and consume plenty of electrolytes! I also recommend the Smart Water brand as the bottles are larger to help you drink more, and it is mineral infused to taste good, too. You can find Smart Water at the best price at the local Costco.

Zero or Low Carb Alcohol is not 100 Percent Keto

Sorry folks, no alcohol for your first 7 Day Challenge week. The reason zero-carb and low-calorie alcohol is not 100 percent Keto-friendly is because of the way our bodies process the liquor.

If you are in ketosis, your body will use fat for energy. When alcohol enters your system, your liver will default to using the byproducts of the metabolized alcohol instead of fat, which means fatty acid oxidation (the process of creating ketones) is slowed until all the alcohol has been processed. Think of alcohol as a fourth (non-essential) macronutrient similar to carbohydrates in that alcohol will halt or slow down fat-burning and ketone production.

Alcohol ties up the liver as it works to detoxify this toxin (I hate that it's a toxin) out of your system. When you drink alcohol, it slows down the production of ketones, which also happens in the liver. Drinking any alcohol can also trigger you to binge on higher-carb foods, which adds insult to injury. Different from carbohydrates, alcohol does not raise blood sugar levels. In moderation, a Keto-friendlier wine or liquor cocktail will not completely de-rail your keto lifestyle. If you enjoy a drink occasionally, plenty of low-carb options can be added to your Keto lifestyle later once you get rolling.

There is a simple and delicious vodka "Keto-Tini" recipe that I included in my free gift to you of my top five favorite Keto comfort food swaps here: https://evanhabits.com/free-recipes/

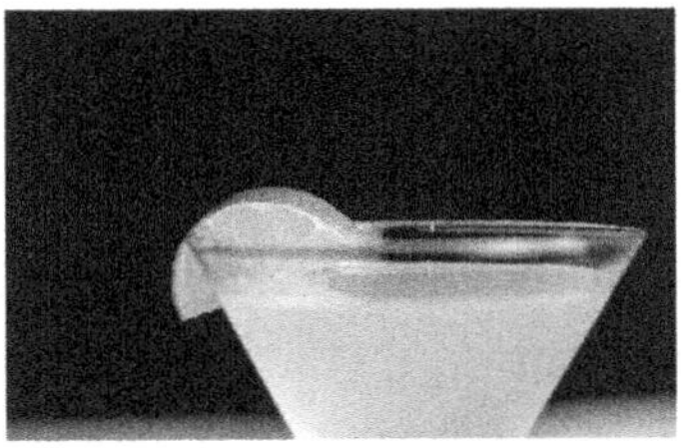

Or scan the Q.R. code by taking a picture from your cell phone camera below:

Where to shop for your Challenge foods?

Wherever the best Keto deals are in your local market! Be sure to join our Challenge Facebook Group as we post *Keto Market*

Finds that we uncover in the major national grocery food marketplaces. We post about new Keto items and really anything Keto we find at a great price, too! I know only some food retailers are in every market, but most of the above retailers are near you or will be soon.

Aldi – Costco - Trader Joe's – Sam's Club – Local health food stores – Farmer's Markets

---

Tracking Your Results: N/1 means your own controlled personal experiment.

How do you really know what is best for YOU?! You need to test it and prove it to yourself. You are doing just that here! This Challenge is your very own N/1 experiment.

It compares the "old you" activity results against the "new you" activity. You will compare your simple keto eating results to your baseline, which is how you were eating before. While conducting this personal keto experiment, you will need to take notice and journal some notes along the way. Never go by a friend or family member's outline for eating the way they do. If it works for them, then... *It works for them.*

Take a "selfie" in your bathing suit of your full body and a close-up of your face before starting your Challenge. Over a short amount of time, you will see your face change and become less full-looking as inflammation goes down in your body and your head. After seven days of eating Keto, compare your before "Carb face" to your after "Keto face" and your full body shot. It may take a few weeks to really see the difference, but it can be dramatic.

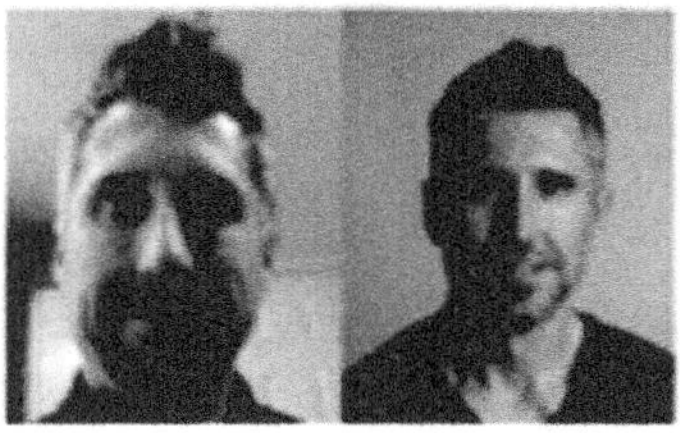

Carb face Keto face

Before you begin your 7 Day Challenge, take the time to put your tightest-fitting pair of jeans on. Notice how they fit (or, more likely, don't fit) and how they make you look and feel before you begin. After seven days of eating Keto, see if they feel any different when you try them on. Plan on donating your "fat pants" to a local non-profit charity soon!

Always journal your results! If you don't track your results, you have nothing to reflect on to see if eating Keto will work for you as a lifestyle upgrade.

Simple daily journal question prompts:

- ❑ *How do I feel?*
- ❑ *How do I look in the mirror?*
- ❑ *Is this way of eating sustainable for me "as is"?*

❏ *How can I tweak this to make it work even better for me next week?*

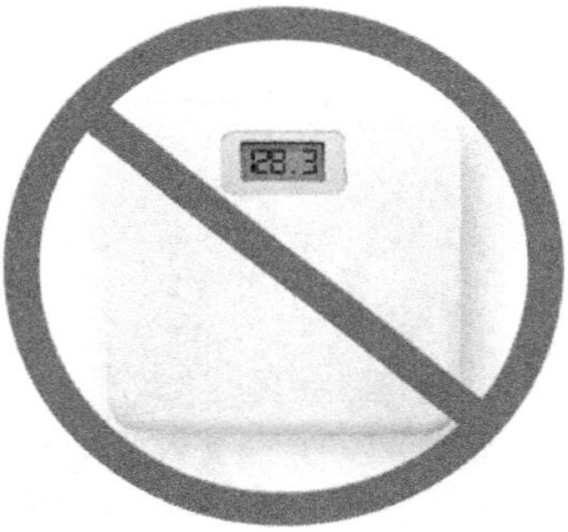

You are not the number on your scale! As a reminder, we are not tracking scale weight here at all or calories, either. It's not about the number on the scale. It's all about how you look and feel, regardless of the number on the scale.

The "Hell Yeah" or "Hard Pass" filter!

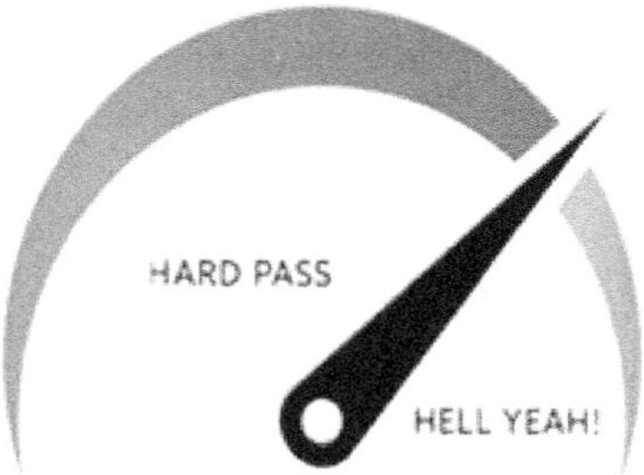

This helpful decision-making filter is based on a scale of 1–10, with 10 being the best. If the thing I am considering doing or eating is not an 8 or higher (eliciting a Hell Yeah! reaction when you consider it), then... it's a Hard Pass. Use this simple filter for a more satisfying life, as it helps you make upgraded decisions about everything, including what you choose to eat! I encourage you to decide to do and eat only the things that move your happiness needle to the right, hard! Life is meant to be enjoyed to the fullest!

Free online tools to keep you organized

Calendar

Google.com - Calendar

Another free tool inside your free Gmail account. Use your calendar to enter your weekly meal plan for each day of the upcoming week. By adding your meals to your calendar, you are making this an "appointment priority" and ensuring it will happen. If you follow your first Challenge week the way it's all set up for you, the grocery list and daily food calendar are 100 percent done for you already. *Minimum Effective Keto.* If you choose to continue eating Keto and want to add/delete meals to personalize the diet more to your taste, just plug those changes into your calendar.

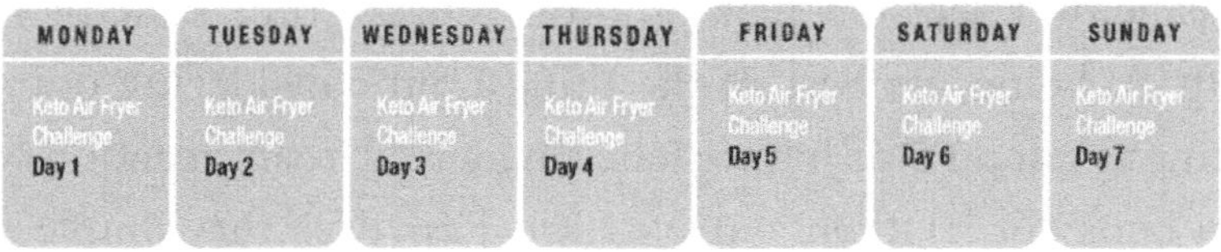
MONDAY
Keto Air Fryer Challenge Day 1
TUESDAY
Keto Air Fryer Challenge Day 2
WEDNESDAY
Keto Air Fryer Challenge Day 3
THURSDAY
Keto Air Fryer Challenge Day 4
FRIDAY
Keto Air Fryer Challenge Day 5
SATURDAY
Keto Air Fryer Challenge Day 6
SUNDAY
Keto Air Fryer Challenge Day 7

Keep

Google.com - Keep app

Another free tool inside the suite of your free Gmail account. This simple app is perfect for entering your Challenge journal notes as you progress through your Challenge week and beyond.

Workflowy

Workflowy.com - Best FREE "to-do list" app

This is an excellent free, organized list-making tool with upgrade options, too. This tool will help you stay on track with just about anything in your life, including but not limited to grocery lists and favorite recipes, and to journal your 7 Day Challenge results. I love this tool, as it has a few more options than the Google Keep tool, and you can share your lists with others. If you struggle with ADHD like I do or just with keeping everything in your life straight, this tool is for you!

- **Recipes 5 stars (must be Hell Yeah! or "Hard Pass")** - simple, tasty, rinse and repeat -Keto Comfort food swaps
    - Instant pot recipes...
    - **FAT (BOO) tea,** water, coffee...shots.
    - coffee line ups - Tom delauer video. (tea idea) FAT water, collagen add. -
    - **Buffalo chicken "nuggets", strips swap** - yes.
    - Bacon as a condiment
    - **Keto cheese sauce recipe**
    - Dressings - creamy avocado cucumber, ________ . ACV is good in any of these...
    - **Buffalo Butter Sauce**- Awesome on Broccoli (Onion powder + Sea Salt)
    - Backing into healthy ingredients - Spinach, broccoli, Kale, romaine, Wheat Grass, cauliflower, celery, ice berg lettuce, cucumber, ACV (dressings), easy-healthy-keto upgrades- FATS how to get healthy fats into recipes easy. (Tom delauer video)
    - Easy Basil Hollandaise sauce recipe - 30 day cleanse book p. ?
    - **GF beef seasoned "Taco Meat" on anything**

***What's Next?* Do this thing!!**

After you follow the first week's Challenge blueprint with the simple Keto recipes from the 7 Day Air Fryer Challenge recipes guide, you will then have a simple choice to make going into week number two and beyond:

Rinse and Repeat

Keep things exactly the same for another week, with still 0 decisions required on your part to keep eating Keto.

Tweak Recipes and Repeat

Swap a few new Keto foods or recipes into the same weekly system you already have for more variety based on your unique tastes and desire to cook.

Refer to www.evanhabits.com and join The Challenge Facebook Group for more Keto recipe ideas and great Keto market deals we come across when shopping to support your Keto lifestyle!

LET'S GET STARTED!!

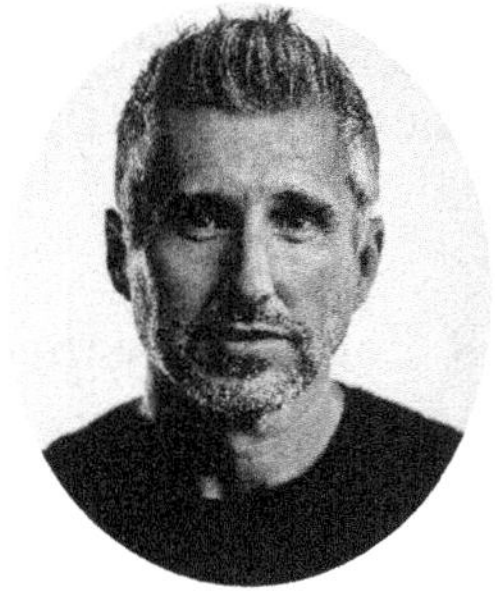

It's never too late to improve how you look and feel. I'm fifty-three now, and I can tell you that after changing my fuel source from sugar to fat about ten years ago, I look and feel better now than in my early twenties. No matter your age, it's just not normal to feel like hot garbage. It doesn't have to be that way for us! Age is just a number, and it alone should not dictate how we feel.

My Challenge when putting this book together for you? How could I get you, my friend, to try Keto or maybe try it again and make it so simple that your results were guaranteed? *It had to be a no-brainer.* It had to be the most straightforward version of the keto diet that has ever been put online in a book or course. I needed to come up with the *Minimum Effective Keto Diet.*

Mission Accomplished.

It's now time for you to DO the thing!! Get your calendar out, and fill in the Monday you will kick off your 7 Day Challenge! Now you have the simple, proven, effective concepts on what to do (and what not do) and the critical "how to" part as well.

"Cheers to your health and happiness!"

The resource page for your 7 Day Keto Air Fryer Challenge is here: https://evanhabits.com/recommended/ I have a page with simple links straight to every product or supplement I recommended in this book on Amazon so that you can order those things if you need them before you begin your Challenge. There are a few more recommendations on other products that I love that you can consider, too.

Use the camera on your phone to scan the Q.R. code below that will get you right to the recommended products page here.

If you have Amazon Prime, it's free shipping to your front door for added convenience.

Also, please join the Challenge Facebook Community, an excellent group full of inspiring, like-minded individuals who are focusing on upgrading their lives through healthy habits, just like you and I right here: https://www.facebook.com/ketolifeupgrade

Use the camera on your phone to scan the Q.R. code below to get you right to the Facebook group page here:

REFERENCES

Interest in the Ketogenic Diet Grows for Weight Loss and Type 2 Diabetes, Abbasi, JAMA, 2018

Meta-analysis of VLCKD vs low-fat diets for long term weight loss, Bueno et al, 2013.

Meta-analysis of low-fat diets vs other diets for long term weight loss, Tobias et al, 2015.

"With too much information," says Dimoka, "people's decisions make less and less sense." Angelika Dimoka, https://www.fox.temple.edu/news/2018/04/research-gets-inside-your-head, 2018

The Science of Making Decisions, https://www.newsweek.com/science-making-decisions-68627, Sharon Begley, 2011

The U.S. News and World Report, https://health.usnews.com/best-diet/best-diets-overall, 2023

Prevalence of Overweight and Obesity adults, https://www.niddk.nih.gov/health-information/health-statistics/overweight-obesity, 2017-2018

The Social Dilemma, https://www.netflix.com/title/81254224, Jeff Orlowski, 2020

https://www.myplate.gov/eat-healthy/what-is-myplate, U.S. Department of Agriculture, 2020-2025, dietary guidelines for Americans, https://www.dietaryguidelines.gov/

Mindless Eating: The 200 Daily Food Decisions We Overlook, Environment and Behavior, Brian Wansink and Jeffery Sobal, 2007

What you need to know about willpower: The psychological science of self-control, American Psychological Association, https://www.apa.org/topics/personality/willpower, 2023

Baumeister, R., & Tierney, J. (2011) *Willpower: Rediscovering the Greatest Human Strength.* New York: Penguin Press.

Danziger, S., Levav, J., & Avnaim-Pesso, L. (2011). *Extraneous factors in judicial decisions.* Proceedings of the National Academy of Sciences,108(17), 6889-6892, https://www.pnas.org/doi/10.1073/pnas.1018033108, 2011

The Paradox of Choice: Why More Is Less. Barry Schwartz, December 2004, Scientific American.

What Is MCT Oil and How Does It Work with the Keto Diet? Amy Richter, Healthline 2019.

Dinicolantonio, J. J., O'Keefe, J. H., & Wilson, W. L. (2018). Sugar addiction: is it real? A narrative review. *Neuroscience & Biobehavioral Reviews, 92,* 526-539. https://doi.org/10.1016/j.neubiorev.2018.05.032

FoodData Central, https://fdc.nal.usda.gov/fdc-app.html#/food-details/168446/nutrients, U.S. Department Of Agriculture, 2018

Are Organic Eggs Worth the Money? Jillian Kubala, Healthline, 2019.

Ketones and Nutritional Ketosis: Basic Terms and Concepts, https://www.virtahealth.com/blog/ketone-ketosis-basics, Stephen Phinney, MD, PhD and Jeff Volek, PhD, R.D., 2018

The Science of Nutritional Ketosis and Appetite, https://www.virtahealth.com/blog/ketosis-appetite-hunger, Stephen Phinney, MD, PhD and Jeff Volek, PhD, R.D., 2018

Murray, A. J., Knight, N. S., Cole, M. A., Cochlin, L. E., Carter, E., Tchabanenko, K., ... & Clarke, K. (2016). Novel ketone diet enhances physical and cognitive performance. *FASEB Journal,* 30(12), 4021-4032.

Lally, P., van Jaarsveld, C. H. M., Potts, H. W. W., & Wardle, J. (2009). How are habits formed: Modelling habit formation in the real world. *European Journal of Social Psychology,* 40(6), 998–1009. https://doi.org/10.1002/ejsp.674

Centers for Disease Control and Prevention (CDC). (2021). *Overweight and Obesity*. Retrieved from https://www.cdc.gov/obesity/data/adult.html

MCT oil benefits, published studies

St-Onge, M. P., Bosarge, A., Goree, L. L. T., & Darnell, B. (2008). Medium chain triglyceride oil consumption as part of a weight loss diet does not lead to an adverse metabolic profile when compared to olive oil. *The American Journal of Clinical Nutrition,* 87(3), 820-827. https://doi:10.1093/ajcn/87.3.820

St-Onge, M. P., Mayrsohn, B., O'Keeffe, M., Kissileff, H. R., Choudhury, A. R., & Laferrère, B. (2014). Impact of medium and long chain triglycerides consumption on appetite and food intake in overweight men. *European Journal of Clinical Nutrition,* 68(10), 1134-1140. https://doi:10.1038/ejcn.2014.145

Reger, M. A., Henderson, S. T., Hale, C., Cholerton, B., Baker, L. D., Watson,

G. S., . . . Craft, S. (2004). Effects of β-hydroxybutyrate on cognition in memory-impaired adults. *Neurobiology of Aging*, 25(3), 311-314. https://doi:10.1016/S0197-4580(03)00087-3

Hertzler, S. R., & Savaiano, D. A. (1996). Colonic adaptation to daily lactose feeding in lactose maldigesters reduces lactose intolerance. *The American Journal of Clinical Nutrition*, 64(2), 232-236. https://doi:10.1093/ajcn/64.2.232

Babayan, V. K. (1987). Medium chain length fatty acid esters and their medical and nutritional applications. *Journal of the American Oil Chemists' Society*, 64(11), 1559-1565. https://doi:10.1007/BF02637101

Exogenous ketone published data references:

Stubbs, B. J., Cox, P. J., Evans, R. D., Santer, P., Miller, J. J., Faull, O. K., ... & Clarke, K. (2018). On the metabolism of exogenous ketones in humans. *Frontiers in Physiology*, 9, 1135.

Cox, P. J., Kirk, T., Ashmore, T., Willerton, K., Evans, R., Smith, A., ... & King, M. T. (2016). Nutritional ketosis alters fuel preference and, thereby endurance performance in athletes. *Cell Metabolism*, 24(2), 256-268.

Krikorian, R., Shidler, M. D., Dangelo, K., Couch, S. C., Benoit, S. C., & Clegg, D. J. (2012). Dietary ketosis enhances memory in mild cognitive impairment. *Neurobiology of Aging*, 33(2), 425-e19.

Kesl, S. L., Poff, A. M., Ward, N. P., Fiorelli, T. N., Ari, C., Van Putten, A. J., ... & D'Agostino, D. P. (2017). Effects of exogenous ketone supplementation on blood ketone, glucose, triglyceride, and lipoprotein levels in Sprague–Dawley rats. *Nutrition & Metabolism*, 14(1), 1-9.

Made in United States
North Haven, CT
03 April 2024

50876283R00078